LEARNING THEORY
APPROACHES TO PSYCHIATRY

LEARNING THEORY APPROACHES TO PSYCHIATRY

Edited by

John C. Boulougouris

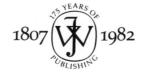

JOHN WILEY & SONS

Chichester · New York · Brisbane · Toronto · Singapore

Library of Congress Cataloging in Publication Data:
Main entry under title:
Learning theory approaches to psychiatry.
    A collection of selected articles presented at the International
Symposium on Learning Theory Approaches to Psychiatry held at
the Orthodox Academy of Crete, April 1980, sponsored by Greek
Ministry of Culture and Science and the Greek Association for
Behaviour Modification and Research.
    Includes indexes.
    1. Behavior therapy—Congresses. 2. Behavior modification—
Congresses. 3. Learning, Psychology of—Congresses.
I. Boulougouris, J. C. II. International Symposium on Learning
Theory Approaches to Psychiatry (1980: Orthodox Academy of
Crete). III. Greece. Hypourgeion Politismou kai Epistēmōn.
IV. Greek Association for Behaviour Modification and Research.

RC489.B4L42   616.89'142   81–16514

ISBN 0 471 28042 9

British Library Cataloguing in Publication Data:
Learning theory approaches to psychiatry.
    1. Psychiatry—Methodology—Congresses
    I. Boulougouris, John C.
    616.8'900'8   RC454.4

ISBN 0 471 28042 9

Typeset by Computacomp (UK) Ltd, Fort William, Scotland
Printed in the United States of America

LIST OF CONTRIBUTORS

Numbers in parentheses indicate the pages on which the authors' contributions begin.

Annable, Lawrence (245). Department of Psychiatry, McGill University, Montreal, Canada.

Barlow, David (75). Department of Psychology, State University of New York at Albany, 1400 Washington Avenue, Albany, New York 12222, USA.

Bloeschl, Lilian (231). Department of Educational Psychology, University of Graz, A 8010 Graz, Hans-Sachs-Casse 3/2, Austria.

Bolsover, Nick (171). Rotheram District General Hospital, Rotheram, South Yorkshire, England.

Borkovec, Thomas (95). Department of Psychology, The Pennsylvania State University, 544 Moore Bldg. University Park, Pa 16802, USA.

Borrmann, Gabriele (219). Heimat für Heimatlose GmbH Coppelrain Sozialpädagogische Einrichtung für Kinder und Jugendliche, Postfach 1106, D-7110 Öhringen. West Germany.

Boulougouris, John (143). Department of Psychiatry, Athens Medical School, Vasilissis Sophias 119, Athens, Greece.

Constantopoulos, Athanassios (111). Psychotherapy Unit, Derbyshire Area Health Authority, 22 Laurie House, Colyear Street, Derby DE1 1BG, England.

Eelen, Paul (3). Department Psychologie, Universiteit te Leuven, Tienestraat 102, Leuven, Belgium.

Emmelkamp, Paul (119). Academic Department of Clinical Psychology, Groningen, The Netherlands.

Everaerd, Walter (165). State University of Utrecht, Trans 4, 3512 JK Utrecht, The Netherlands.

Florin, Irmela (219). Fachbereich Psychologie der Philipps-Universität Marburg, D-3500 Marburg/Lahn Gutenbergstrasse 18, West Germany.

Foa, Edna (129). Department of Psychiatry, Temple University School of Medicine, Eastern Pennsylvania Psychiatric Institute, Henry Ave. Philadelphia, Pa 19129, USA.

Garelis, Evangelos (237). Department of Psychiatry, Eginition Hospital, Vasilissis Sophias 74, Athens, Greece.

Gelder, Michael (87). Department of Psychiatry, University of Oxford, Warneford Hospital, Oxford OX3 7JX, England.

Grayson, Jonathan (129). Department of Psychiatry, Temple University School of Medicine, Eastern Pennsylvania Psychiatric Institute, Henry Ave. Philadelphia, Pa 19129, USA.   -

Herbert, Martin (191). Child Treatment Research Unit, School of Social Work, University of Leicester, 107 Princess Road East, Leicester LE1 7LA, England.

Jardine, Yvonne (111). University of Leeds, Department of Psychiatry, Leeds (St James's) University Hospital, Leeds, England.

Katkin, Edward (67). Department of Psychology, State University of New York at Buffalo, 4230 Ridge Lea Road, Buffalo, New York 14226, USA.

Kockott, Götz (171). Max-Planck-Institut für Psychiatrie, Kraepelinstrasse 10, 800 München 40, West Germany.

Lavallée Yvon-Jacques (245). Maisonneuve-Rosemont Hospital and Department of Psychiatry, Université de Montreal, Montreal, Canada.

Lamontagne, Yves (245). Research Unit, Louis-H. Lafontaine Hospital and Department of Psychiatry, Université de Montreal, Montreal, Canada.

Liappas, John (143). Department of Psychiatry, Eginition Hospital, Vasilissis Sophias 74, Athens, Greece.

Mathews, Andrew (157). Department of Psychology, St George's Hospital Medical School, University of London, Jenner Wing, Crammer Terrace, London SW17, England.

Marks, Isaac (19). Institute of Psychiatry, University of London, De Crespigny Park, Denmark Hill, London SE5 8AF, England.

Melamed, Barbara (205). Department of Clinical Psychology, University of Florida, Gainesville, 32610 USA.

Pfäfflin, Friedemann (179). Abteilung für Sexualforschung, der Universät Hamburg, Martinistrasse 52, 2000 Hamburg 20, West Germany.

Rabavilas, Andreas (143). Department of Psychiatry, Eginition Hospital, Vasilissis Sophias 74, Athens, Greece.

Ross, Jerilyn (103). The Phobia Programme of Washington, 6191 Executive Boulevard, Rockville, Maryland 20852, USA.

Schimikowski, Cornelia (219). Zum Raumwäldchen 8, D-5902 Netphen 1, West Germany.

Snaith, Philip (111). University of Leeds, Department of Psychiatry, Leeds (St James's) University Hospital, Leeds, England.

Steketee, Gail (129). Department of Psychiatry, Temple University School of Medicine, Eastern Pennsylvania Psychiatric Institute, Henry Ave. Philadelphia, Pa 19129, USA.

Tabouratzis, Dimitri (143). Laskarithou 10–14, Kalithea, Athens, Greece.

Teasdale, John (57). Department of Psychiatry, University of Oxford Warneford Hospital, Oxford OX3 7JK, England.

Wilson, G. Terence (33). Department of Psychology, Rutgers, The State University of New Jersey, Busch. Campus. P.O. Box 819, Piscataway, New Jersey 08854, USA.

CONTENTS

PREFACE

The Greek Association for Behaviour Modification and Research, a multidisciplinary body of people interested in promoting the advancement of learning principles in behaviour modification, organized in Crete on April 12–16, 1980, an International Symposium on 'Learning Theory Approaches to Psychiatry'. Eminent investigators from various countries were brought together and discussions centred on theoretical issues regarding the relevance of learning theories to behavioural therapies. Papers giving an up-to-date account of clinical research in the treatment of neurotic and behavioural disorders were also presented.

Most participants' contributions were outstanding and threw some more light onto the inadequacies and limitations of the thus far developed theoretical conceptualizations for explaining the effectiveness of various behavioural approaches applied on psychiatric patients. The participants' response convinced me that this symposium would contribute to our field and therefore I undertook the difficult and challenging task of publishing these proceedings. The theoretical considerations related to the mechanisms of action of treatment procedures, the new theoretical formulations put forward, and the wealth of clinical research data presented in this volume should enable theoreticians and clinical research workers to acquire a better grasp of the current trends concerning the applications of behavioural principles to psychopathological conditions, and stimulate further research for the development of a unified psychological theory and improvement of the present therapeutic strategies.

This symposium was sponsored by the Greek Ministry of Culture and Science and our Association gratefully acknowledges this support. I would like to thank all members of the symposium committee for their help and in particular the staff and Alexandros Papaderos of the Orthodox Academy of Crete where the symposium took place and which provided all the facilities for the gathering. The editor would also like to thank the contributors to this volume who have met the publication demands without complaint and his wife, Jennifer, for editorial and other assistance.

JOHN C. BOULOUGOURIS
Athens Medical School

INTRODUCTION

This volume is a collection of selected articles presented at the International Symposium on 'Learning Theory Approaches to Psychiatry' held in Crete, in April of 1980. Since learning theory is at present inadequate to explain the genesis and maintenance of psychotic behaviour, this symposium did not deal with treatment procedures modifying such behaviour. We were concerned almost exclusively with neurotic disorders treated with therapeutic interventions based mainly on learning principles, bearing in mind that learning theory is still at its frontiers when explaining neurotic behaviour. Twenty-three chapters, in six parts, were written by research workers, experts in a particular field, and as editor in this introductory chapter I will make some general orienting comments and briefly outline the main points of each contribution.

The first part of the volume, which contains six chapters, is concerned with the main and most controversial topic of the symposium: *Relationship of Learning Theory to Behavioural Therapies*. Such a topic was chosen as the main theme due to the increasing dissatisfaction with existing learning theories in explaining the psychopathology and mechanisms of action of almost all behavioural techniques. On the other hand, the evidence gathered so far has shown that the effectiveness of most behavioural techniques on several psychological disorders cannot be disputed. However, techniques which for years had been considered effective, were later proved ineffective. Our memories are still fresh from the treatment of obesity by attaching electrodes to the spoon or fork, and delivering shocks to homosexuals and alcoholics. Our previous enthusiasm and confidence was shaken by well-designed studies which showed that the successful application of some techniques may be due to the possible contribution of non-specific or placebo effects. The notion that 'the relief of a mental patient from his discomfort is what matters' regardless of how the treatment works and regardless of any theoretical framework, is dangerous and leads to more confusion which will probably create disastrous consequences in the near future. We are all aware that the Watson and the Miller–Mowrer conditioning models were very influential and fundamental to our thinking and practice in behaviour therapy although they were not fulfilling as proper theoretical systems. Seligman's notion of 'preparedness' is of great value for understanding at least the phobic reactions and explaining the lack of equipotentiality. Furthermore, Gray's model, the significance of 'uncertainty' as the basic UCS in the development of anxiety, the theory of the incubation of anxiety, and the 'cognitive theory' approach, all attempt to give alternative explanations of the genesis and maintenance of neurotic behaviour. The strong criticism over behaviourism, particularly by the 'cognitive theory' advocates and vice versa, do not seem to have stimulated researchers and theorists into creative thinking in order to fill our present theoretical gaps and throw more light on the underlying processes in most behavioural techniques. Nevertheless, the first chapter of Part One provides an outstanding contribution towards a constructive synthesis, instead of using argumentative academic exercises, wherein Eelen reviews the impact of Garcia-effect on psychological theories and proposes that a strong link between conditioning and attribution might be a step towards understanding how a behaviour is acquired and maintained. In this context, unconscious processes may have their merit, a view which is not shared by most behaviour therapists. He also suggests that classical conditioning is not just an automatic process but an active information process and that a machinery for this purpose lies within the organism. The importance of the similarity and spatial contiguity of events to be associated is stressed and taste aversion seems to be a central memory phenomenon. He concludes that the dichotomy of learning and cognition has not been proved fruitful and the integration of current theories, without forgetting Pavlov's dog, within our therapeutic endeavours is needed. Marks, in Chapter Two, supports the view that conditioning language is unsatisfactory to explain the phenomenology of phobias and rituals. He reviews thoroughly the important experiments on prepotency, preparedness and differential conditioning, and he suggests that terms more closely tied to the clinical phenomena such as evoking stimuli, response decrement, should be adopted in order to elaborate more satisfactory models for psychopathology and will have more practical value. Wilson, in Chapter Three, stresses from the beginning the importance of being theoretical and that theoretical developments have lagged behind the general growth of behaviour therapy. His contribution is an extensive review of almost all existing learning theories but particular emphasis is given to the alternative theoretical frameworks which have been developed over the past decade. Most attention is given to Bandura's social learning and self-efficacy theories by pointing out their contribution to the continuing growth of behaviour therapies. However, the failure to find significant correlation between efficacy expectations and either self-reports or physiological measures of fear arousal and the inconsistent findings regarding the power of efficacy expectations limit the support of self-efficacy theory. Bio-informational theory of emotional imagery with the triple response system analysis of behaviour as formulated by Lang is another promising advance in our knowledge of behaviour change and the author foresees that for the future, at least in United States, that more emphasis will be given to technological development within the field. Teasdale attempts to answer the most difficult question of what needs to be done for us to acquire better understanding of psychopathology and how more effective therapeutic procedures can be developed. He proposes in Chapter Four that a theory is needed which should provide an integrated account of the maintainance of a psychiatric condition we wish to treat and of the means of treating it. He also points out that a theory which is paradigm-related and with empirical support is more likely to give an answer to the question of improving psychological treatment. The relationship of learning and biofeedback, a promising therapeutic tool for behavioural medicine and psychiatry in the 1970s, is discussed in Chapter Five by Katkin. After defining the distinction between an active treatment effect and a placebo effect, he supports, as do most researchers in his field, the belief that effective control of autonomic functions requires the establishment of response reinforcement contingencies. On the other hand, he argues that the history of biofeedback research is characterized by a dreary record of poorly controlled studies. He actually attributes this inadequacy to the lack of having a sound conceptual base for the analysis of placebo effects and therefore the contribution of non-specific variables to the therapeutic outcome is still an open question. Although Barlow in Chapter Six realizes that learning and pure conditioning principles will never be sufficient in treating various psychiatric problems, he tries to support the notion that conditioning is an important ingredient at least in aversion and covert sensitization techniques. He actually presents some data on four patients with undesired sexual arousal who undergo treatment by covert sensitization, and shows that expectancies or rehearsing the aversive stimulus in a self-control fashion have little to do with the outcome.

The next four chapters of Part Two are devoted to the *Treatment of Phobic Disorders*. The investigation of fear responses and of phobias were the most favourable research areas by learning theorists, experimenters, and behaviour therapists over the past few decades. The fruitful outcome of this enormous research work is reflected today by the successful application of behavioural techniques in clinical practice. However, we are still far away from understanding phobias and most questions regarding the underlying processes of various treatment procedures are left unanswered. Although exposure-based methods have been shown to be the most effective interventions for the majority of agoraphobic patients, Gelder in Chapter Seven questions the necessity and the sufficiency of exposure in such patients. After a brief description of the so-called programmed practice treatment for agoraphobics, developed in Oxford over the past few years, he compares this treatment with a control (problem-solving) treatment, and in his elegant study he shows the superiority of programmed practice which gives emphasis to exposure to the feared situations. However, evidence derived from this investigation indicates that exposure itself is of little value if it is not combined with anxiety management techniques and change of attitude regarding helplessness. Furthermore, his results suggest that exposure may not be a necessary condition for improvement since patients improved when they became less anxious and more confident. Borkovec in Chapter Eight examines almost the same question as Gelder but from another perspective in order to explain what the phobic patient does to prevent the occurrence of CS exposure, despite the objective presentation of the fear stimuli in real life or during therapy. He assumes that phobics reduce awareness of or attention to the phobic stimuli and the effect of internal cues in maintaining avoidance behaviour is of paramount importance. Apart from the *in vivo* exposure techniques currently applied on such patients, he shows that expectancy and relaxation may facilitate functional CS exposure, as extinction is taking place via the reduction of cognitive avoidance. On the other hand, the paradoxical effect of relaxation on generally anxious clients attributed to the internal nature of CS in clients is discussed. The role of the spouse or other family member in the exposure treatment with phobic patients is presented by Ross in Chapter Nine. She illustrates the verbal interaction between a family member and a phobic patient during the practice session and comments on three cases showing the important role of the family member in the therapy. Finally, in Chapter Ten Constantopoulos and his colleagues, in an unfinished project, investigate the therapeutic programme of 'Anxiety Control Training' with and without instructions for exposure to threatening situations for phobic patients. They show that exposure to focalized anxiety does not improve short-term outcome and discuss the results gathered so far from the point of view of Banduras theory of 'self-efficacy'.

The fourth part of this volume deals with the *Treatment of Obsessive Compulsive Disorders*. The treatment of choice at least for the non-depressed obsessive–compulsive patients appears to be exposure and response prevention. The advantages of exposure in the home environment and the beneficial effects of involving family members in the therapy have been stressed by researchers in this area. The therapeutic efficacy of exposure seems to be enhanced by training patients in decision making and problem solving approaches whereas depressed obsessive–compulsives are benefited by Clomipramine. 'Pure' obsessionals on the other hand, are very difficult to treat and there is still a number of non-responders to exposure. The processes operating on exposure treatment also remain obscure as in phobias. So, Emmelkamp in Chapter Eleven reviews the recent advances in the treatment of obsessive–compulsive disorders and based on the clinical observations that obsessive–compulsive patients are often socially anxious and unassertive, he shows the results of a case study in which assertive-training is compared to self-controlled exposure *in vivo*. The greater effect of assertive training in reducing obsessive–compulsive pathology is shown, giving less grounds to the anxiety reduction hypothesis regarding the function of obsessive–compulsive rituals. However, such findings need to be replicated as not all obsessive–compulsive patients are unassertive and maybe this type of treatment is suitable for a particular type of patient. Foa and her coworkers in Chapter Twelve examine the relationship between depression, habituation and treatment outcome. The data presented confirm clinical observations that severely depressed obsessive–compulsives do not respond to exposure and response prevention treatment as favourably as non-depressed patients. Regarding the effect of habituation on outcome, it is shown that intra-session habituation is not a sufficent condition for symptom reduction and that the relationship between depression and habituation is mediated by a high level of anxiety associated with depression. Undoubtedly the latter finding needs to be substantiated as possibly orientating us to the use of other techniques on patients with high level of reported anxiety. Since the process underlying exposure is still unclear, Boulougouris and his associates in Chapter Thirteen, look at the importance of the therapeutic relationship and the therapists' variables on outcome in phobic and obsessive–compulsive patients treated with exposure *in vivo*. Comparing experienced and inexperienced therapists whilst they were applying the same exposure method the authors could not find outcome differences between therapists. Phobics and obsessive–compulsive patients responded similarly to both type of therapists. Taking into consideration the intrinsically difficult factors in undertaking research on these lines, it is suggested that better clarification of the concepts used in defining the patient–therapist relationship and the incorporation of communication variblespivariables in future research are needed before definite conclusions can be reached.

Since the publication in 1970 of Masters and Johnson's *Human Sexual Inadequacy* sex therapy and research have been expanded to such an extent that an increasing number of thoughtful researchers in behaviour therapy have diverted their interest and practice towards this area. Such diversion of interest is really justified as the success rates of sex therapy application to sexual problems are far better than any other type of behaviour therapy administered on neurotic disorders. Part Four of this volume deals with the new developments in the *Treatment of Sexual Disorders* beginning with Mathews in Chapter Fourteen where the traditional concept of anxiety inhibiting sexual responding is challenged. In order to clarify some of the factors involved in the treatment of female sexual dysfunction, he presents some data from an ongoing project in which the factors, one versus two therapists, monthly versus weekly sessions and testosterone versus placebo, were tested. It is shown that all these factors are not associated with differences in outcome. However, it can be concluded that the anxiety reduction hypothesis is not the treatment mechanism, anxiolytic medication has a rather negative effect and nothing concrete can be said yet regarding the aetiology of loss of sexual interest in women. Some psychological characteristics and possible psychopathological processes operating on males with different sexual complaints are discussed by Everaerd in Chapter Fifteen. He also refers to an ongoing project comparing sex therapy to Rational Emotive Therapy, pointing out the high rate of drop-outs between male complainants. This finding brings to surface the crucial variables involved in any successful treatment such as motivation, emotional interaction, low sexual desire, and sexual aversion, and the author gives more attention to orientation of feelings in defining sex than to coitus and orgasm as in previous years. Based on the beneficial effects of imitation learning and the impact of a communication setting for a behaviour change Kockott illustrates in Chapter Sixteen how groups of individual patients without partners were treated successfully together with couples. The therapy is mainly behaviourally orientated and he regards that the number of sessions should be limited. Sex education is still needed even for the *young* patients and extensive therapy manual guides for therapists with instructions should be given in order to clarify which type of group is helped most. Almost all research workers in the field of couple sex therapy deliberately avoid taking psychiatric patients with sexual problems for therapy. The exception has arrived from the Department of Sex Research in Hamburg. In Chapter Seventeen Friedmann Plafflin summarizes the methodology employed, the various forms of therapy administered, and the results of a research project on couple therapy carried out from 1972 to 1979. He also takes the opportunity to describe really extraordinary case histories of couples with psychiatric dysfunctions treated successfully. His optimistic message is that psychotic or severely handicapped psychiatric patients with impaired sexual function could show improvement with sex couple therapy which in the past was considered a contraindication.

The fifth part of this volume includes papers related to *Learning Theory and Management of Children's Disorders*. Children's psychopathology is indeed better understood in terms of learning than adulthood behaviour and this is why this topic was selected for discussion in this symposium. The factors involved in shaping the adult's behaviour are so illusive and perplexed that learning alone is inadequate for giving a comprehensive explanation. Herbert in Chapter Eighteen highlights the potential value of the triadic model used at the Child Treatment Research Unit in Leicester for hyperactive children with conduct disorders. The wide choice methods applied to 'home settings' which are based on behaviour modification procedures provide us with very interesting results and the author discusses in length the framework of his work with the families of hyperactive children. Melamed in Chapter Nineteen reviews the research on the psychological preparation of children who are facing stressful medical procedures. The methodological shortcomings in this area of research are mainly attributed to neglect in following the three system approach in defining anxiety. Some data from her recent studies are presented in which film modelling effectiveness is replicated. Investigating the autonomic response patterns of children during exposure to a film indicates that the extent of modelling film intervention in reducing medical stress is determined both by the autonomic arousal property of the film and by the information about treatment that is communicated. In Chapter Twenty Bormann and her colleagues present an analogue study in which the effects of various methods of assertiveness training in children are compared. They show that all experimental groups with the treatment component of active role play present, proved to be superior to the control group. Variables such as motivation, level of anxiety, and sex, seem not to contribute to the differential effects but since their study is analogue one, a similar investigation with clinical population is indicated before any definite conclusion is drawn.

Finally, under *Miscellaneous*, part six of this volume contains two chapters which do not fit into any of the above mentioned parts and another one which seems to be irrelevant to behaviour therapy. In Chapter Twenty-one, Bloeschl discusses the role of psychosocial stressful events and the lack of positive reinforcers in the development of depression. She also suggests that methods based on reinforcement orientated approaches and decrease of aversive stressful events should be used in behavioural modification of depression. Lamontagne and his associates in Chapter Twenty-three deal with the effectiveness of EMG training in the treatment of anxiety and give emphasis to the overall treatment plan of anxiety in which EMG feedback should be used only as an adjuncts to behavioural or insight psychotherapy. In

Chapter Twenty-two, Garelis presents an up-to-date review of drug treatment in obsessive–compulsive disorders. His contribution was considered as appropriate to be included in this volume because readers of such a book are mainly researchers, clinical psychologists and psychiatrists focusing on learning principles to change behaviour and who therefore should find recent information on this topic, looking from another perspective, valuable.

I. RELATIONSHIP OF LEARNING THEORY TO BEHAVIOURAL THERAPIES

Learning Theory Approaches to Psychiatry
Edited by John Boulougouris
© 1982 John Wiley & Sons Ltd

1. CONDITIONING AND ATTRIBUTION

Paul Eelen

Psychology has just celebrated its first centennial. It can be fascinating to read the writings of the early pioneers and, at the same time, it is instructive to remember that the questions which stimulated their research are still with us. The subject of this chapter is related to the seminal work of one of these pioneers: Pavlov and his classical conditioning paradigm. One needs hardly emphasize the importance of Pavlov's work but maybe the time has come for it to be re-emphasized.

The conditioned reaction, elicited by the term 'classical conditioning', is definitely an image of the schematic representation which can be found in almost all introductory textbooks. It can be summarized by four terms: a neutral stimulus will become a *conditioned stimulus*, evoking a *conditioned reaction* if it is presented in a close temporal relation with an *unconditioned stimulus*, evoking spontaneously an *unconditioned reaction* (see Figure 1).

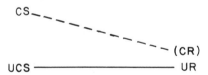

Figure 1. Schematic representation of Pavlovian conditioning

This schematic representation has done a great deal of harm to the appreciation of the significance of Pavlov's original findings. Especially since within this representation are many restrictive conditions. The conditioned stimulus has to be 'neutral' with regard to the unconditioned stimulus, i.e. it is not spontaneously evoking an identical reaction as the unconditioned stimulus. The latter has to be a stimulus spontaneously evoking a well-defined reaction. For this reason, most unconditioned stimuli are of biological significance for the organism. The resulting conditioned reaction is usually identified with some autonomic reaction one of those evoked by the unconditioned stimulus. At the same time, this schematic representation identifies the necessary (and sufficient) condition for conditioning to take place: the temporal contiguity of both stimuli. Finally, this schematic representation identifies learning with a changed reaction towards the CS. Put simply: the dog learns to salivate when he hears the bell ringing.

One has to realize that all these restrictions result from a strong reduction of the original observations. Pavlov's interest in what he called the 'psychic reflex' originated from observing a dog salivating when it heard and saw a man bringing its daily food. This complex event—someone bringing food—has been reduced to a visual or auditive stimulus signalizing food. The event—receiving food—was reduced from seeing a piece of meat in a bowl to meat-powder immediately in the mouth of the dog. And finally, the dog's global reaction was reduced to drops of saliva. This autonomic reaction was of most interest to Pavlov, a physiologist. But after all, it is only one possible index of learning and need not be included in a definition of classical conditioning. 'If conditioning were confined to what some have called "spit and twitches", it would lose much of its psychological interest.' (Rescorla and Holland, 1976, p. 184).

By identifying classical conditioning with this restrictive description, one is hardly surprised to read that the whole paradigm is out of date. Especially within the field of behaviour therapy, the number of 'malcontents'—to paraphrase Wolpe—is growing. The time of Watson seems far behind us. He claimed that the classical conditioning paradigm was the solution for explaining everything in objective terms. We may consider it as scientific progress that nobody still believes Watson's dogmatic claim, but at the same time, our science has progressed by demonstrating that classical conditioning is not so simple and mechanistic as was first thought.

In the first section of this chapter, a summary of some recent findings within the study of classical conditioning will be given. The conclusion will be that classical conditioning involves the study of how an organism learns a relation between at least two events. In the second section, some special inter-event relation will be described: the taste-aversion paradigm. Finally, in the third section, a rather speculative idea is formulated: from the preceding sections, one has to conclude that there is a strong link between conditioning research and attribution theory. Right from the beginning, I want to emphasize that some of these ideas are speculative in the true sense of the word, i.e. they are not very clear to me either.

CLASSICAL CONDITIONING: INTER-EVENT LEARNING

Each organism has to be selectively sensitive to significant and accidental coincidences between events in its environment. Therefore, it is amazing that mere temporal coincidence of two events has been regarded for such a long time as a necessary and even sufficient condition for learning to take place. Recent research findings have clearly demonstrated that this temporal contiguity is neither sufficient nor necessary. From these findings, it becomes clear that conditioning cannot be regarded simply as a matter of registering coincident events. 'If it were, our task as psychologists trying to understand conditioning might be simpler, but our subjects'

success in understanding the world they live in would be very much poorer.'
(Mackintosh, 1978, p. 172). Let us summarize some of these findings. They will
demonstrate how conditioning is dependent upon a rather sophisticated information-
processing capacity of a living organism.

The role of contingency

Coincidence of two events can also be expressed in terms of contingency or
correlation. By using these terms, one wants to emphasize not only the temporal, but
also the logical relation between two events (Rescorla and Holland, 1976). A typical
Pavlovian conditioning experiment arranges not only that the CS is followed by the
US closely in time, but also that the US does not occur frequently, within the given
context, without the CS. Seligman *et al.* (1971) have introduced this idea by drawing
what they call 'the Pavlovian conditioning space' (see Figure 2).

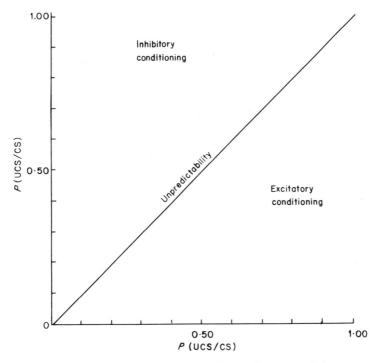

Figure 2.   The Pavlovian conditioning space. The ordinate and abcissa represent the
relationships between CS and UCS. They are stimulus contingencies arranged by the
experimenter. The 45° line represents a special condition, the unpredictability of
Pavlovian reinforcement, because $p(UCS/CS) = p(UCS/\overline{CS})$. Adapted and
reproduced with permission from Seligman *et al.*, *Aversive conditioning and
learning*, Brush (ed.) 1971

In a Pavlovian conditioning experiment, the experimenter has perfect control over the presentation of the two events within this 'conditioning space'. Therefore, it is an excellent paradigm to study the sensitivity of the organism to such correlative relations. Rescorla (1968) initiated many empirical studies on this problem. He demonstrated how the animal was sensitive to the various correlations between CS and US (from perfect positive to perfect negative correlation). In this way, Rescorla has succeeded in translating the two most important Pavlovian findings into contingency-terms: excitatory and inhibitory relations between events. Excitatory conditioning results from learning that two events tend to occur together, inhibitory conditioning results from learning that two events do not occur together.

The necessity of this contingency-relation between two events gives an indication of the fact that 'mere coincidence' is insufficient. The organism is sensitive for the real predictive cues in his environment. From what follows, it will be clear that even 'mere contingency' is insufficient.

Overshadowing

When two stimuli A and B can be used separately as conditioned stimuli, presenting them both together may sometimes result in the conditioning of only one of them. This phenomenon was discussed by Pavlov who introduced the concept of 'saliency' of stimuli, determined by their modality and intensity. In most formal models of classical conditioning, this saliency factor is built in as a parameter of conditioning.

Latent Inhibition and US pre-exposure

Lubow (1973) has introduced the term 'latent inhibition' to label the following observation: pre-exposed stimuli are less effective as signals in subsequent Pavlovian conditioning situations. For instance, if a tone is presented repeatedly by itself and subsequently followed by an electric shock, the organism has difficulty in discovering the signal-value of the tone. It is not clear whether one has to rely on associative or non-associative factors to explain this phenomenon. On the one hand, one may assume that the organism is no longer attending to the stimulus at the moment when it is presented as a signal for something else. On the other hand, the organism may have learned that the stimulus is irrelevant and it has some difficulty in realizing that just this stimulus becomes a signal for something important. In this way, there is a close resemblance between latent inhibition and pre-exposure of the US. If one presents a series of shocks, followed by a sequence of tone preceding shock, it will take a long time before the tone acquires any signalling function. Also in this case, one can rely on associative or non-associative principles as was recently argued by Randich and Lolordo (1979).

Blocking

One of the most convincing demonstrations of the complexity of classical conditioning is Kamin's blocking experiment (Kamin, 1969). This phenomenon has received a lot of attention within the conditioning literature (Mackintosh, 1978). In the basic experimental demonstration, rats are conditioned to a compound CS, consisting of two equally salient elements, A and B, paired with the delivery of a shock as the US. Conditioning is measured by the suppression of on-going appetitively rewarded lever pressing when the CS is presented. Control animals normally show marked suppression to either A or B when they are presented alone; but animals previously conditioned to one of the stimuli alone as a signal for shock show little or no suppression to the other after compound training. For instance, after initial conditioning to A alone in Stage 1, a series of compound trials in Stage 2 during which A and B are repeatedly paired with shock may produce no evidence that B has been associated with the shock. There is at this moment sufficient evidence to defend the position that the organism is attending to stimulus B but, somehow, arrives at the conclusion that it provides irrelevant or at least redundant information with regard to the US.

Conclusion

Even from this brief summary, it becomes clear that the mere coincidence of two events is not a sufficient condition for the learning of a relation between two events. These findings may provide new insight into the whole phenomenon. Instead of an automatic process within a passive organism, classical conditioning seems to postulate an active information-processing organism. Maybe the most important finding is the role of contingency. 'It is one thing, however, to say that the information-processing machinery that an organism brings to the world is designed to be sensitive to contingent relations rather than to coincidentally occurring events. But this tells us relatively little about the exact nature of that machinery. We know, it is true, that we can reject any theory which seeks to reduce conditioning to a simple matter of associating all paired events. But we do not necessarily know what to put in its place.' (Mackintosh, 1978, p. 173). Some authors do not hesitate to assume than an animal has some kind of primitive representation of the so-called contingency-space (Alloy and Seligman, 1979). Others are more careful in making such assumptions. To quote Rescorla: 'Most of us are not comfortable with the notion that organisms take in large blocks of time, count up numbers of US events, and somehow arrive at probability estimates ... It is tempting to think of simple "tricks" that the organism would use to perform in this apparently rational fashion' (Rescorla, 1969, pp. 84–85). In other words, being influenced by a correlative relation between events, does not imply that the organism has any 'idea' of the correlation at all. Therefore, it is remarkable that Rescorla, the champion of the contingency viewpoint, has constructed a theory which essentially goes back to very simple mechanisms (Rescorls and Wagner, 1972). Without going into the details of the formalization of the theory, the basic intuition is simple ans has many implications. As soon as something important happens to the organism which was unexpected, it seems that it tries to find a predictor for this event. This 'discrepancy' seems to be a necessary condition in order for a stimulus to become a signal for this event. As soon as the event has been predicted, either by the general context (US pre-exposure) or by other signals (blocking), no learning takes place. Or to formulate it more exactly: no behavioural evidence of learning can be deduced. This discrepancy notion also explains inhibitory conditioning: if, within a given context, an organism expects too much, the chances are high that this context (or stimulus) becomes inhibitory. It is clear that within this theory, a central role is attributed as well to the global context as to the previous history of the organism.

Intentionally, we have been using metaphors such as 'trying to find a predictor', 'expectation discrepancy', etc. The use of such a vocabulary becomes even more necessary when we have to describe a particular instance of inter-event learning, namely taste aversion which has become popular under the name of the Garcia effect.

TASTE AVERSION: THE GARCIA EFFECT

Maybe the best way to introduce the taste aversion paradigm is 'the sauce béarnaise' phenomenon, described by Seligman and Hager (1972). The night after a dinner with filet-mignon and sauce béarnaise, Seligman became sick. Later on, it became clear that the illness was most probably due to the beginning of 'flu' but Seligman had already 'attributed' it to the sauce béarnaise. Since then, he strongly dislikes the taste of this sauce. Some questions are raised by this anecdote. Why was the illness 'attributed' to the sauce béarnaise and not to other available cues. Why did the aversion not disappear when *post hoc* the beginning of 'flu was a much more plausible cause. Why has the taste of sauce béarnaise since then really become a bad taste?

The same kind of questions are raised by Garcia's findings. In 1966, Garcia and Koelling published a two-page article which, in retrospect, was the beginning of a whole new research paradigm. They demonstrated that rats can easily associate the taste of food with artificially induced 'sickness' but not with shock, whereas for audio-visual stimuli, correlated with food intake, it is just the opposite. These stimuli do not become aversive when they are followed by sickness but they become aversive when shock is contingent upon them. In Pavlovian terms, this finding can be formulated as an interaction between the nature of the US and the nature of the CS. Another important characteristic of Garcia's findings was that taste aversion can be learned even with a long delay between food intake and induced sickness.

At first glance, these findings contradicted the traditional framework of conditioning theories wherein it was always more or less implicitly assumed that general laws of learning can be formulated by taking into account only the extrinsic, experimentally arranged, temporal relations between two (or more) events. Stated in its most primitive form, this assumption of equipotentiality (Seligman, 1970) holds that in order for two events to become associated, one has only to arrange some external temporal relation between them. In other words, temporal contiguity is a necessary and sufficient condition for learning to take place. Apparently, the Garcia effect demonstrated that this temporal contiguity is neither sufficient nor necessary. Intrinsic relations between two events seem to interact with extrinsic relations (Rescorla and Holland, 1976).

The Garcia effect has received a lot of attention, maybe partly due to a provocative article by Seligman (1970) wherein the notion of 'preparedness' was introduced. According to preparedness theory, associations for a certain species can be ordered along a continuum of preparedness, defined in terms of ease of learning. This continuum is based on the assumption that evolutionary contingencies have prepared species to learn easily some things rather than others. Such prepared associations are very rapidly acquired, highly resistant to extinction and minimally affected by cognitive variables. Therefore, they are probably based on a different physiological substrate. The questions raised by Seligman, using the Garcia effect as a prototype of preparedness, have stimulated research into two main directions. One direction, most explicitly represented by Rozin and Kalat (1972), has stressed the importance of viewing learning as part of the organism's whole adaptation to its environment. Therefore, knowledge about the function of learning for a particular species in its natural habitat is much more important than the search for so-called general laws of learning. Viewing learning as part of behavioural biology, this direction of research has brought experimental psychologists and ethologists together. The other direction of research is centred around the question of mechanisms behind so-called prepared learning. For instance, is prepared learning a learning or a performance phenomenon? What specific associative factors characterize prepared associations? Are these phenomena only exceptional to traditional viewpoints because one has only taken into account the temporal relations between events, not paying attention to other factors such as stimulus similarity, spatial relations, temporal intensity patterns, etc. (Testa, 1974, 1975). In other words, within this last direction of research, one is more concerned with explaining the rather exceptional findings by taking into account well-known but less studied factors influencing the learning of a relation between two events.

From this last direction of research, it is becoming clear that taste aversion can be integrated into the general study of how an organism learns a relation between two events (Logue, 1979). All the informational variables which have been described in the first section of this chapter as influencing this learning, seem to be important for learning a taste aversion. First, the role of contingency. A positive contingency has to be arranged between the taste and induced illness. If both events are presented randomly, no aversion is learned. With a negative contingency, a taste preference is created. Also, latent inhibition seems important: if the rat has tasted a solution several times before it is made ill, no taste aversion seems to occur. Also, pre-exposing the rat to illness makes it difficult afterwards to use this illness as a US in a taste aversion experiment. Finally, blocking has been demonstrated too: learning an aversion to one taste can block the learning of an aversion towards another taste. In this context a study by Rudy *et al.* (1977) needs to be mentioned. They first introduced a contingency between an external stimulus, a 'black cage' and illness. When later on the taste of saccharine was introduced within this contingency, the rats did not develop a taste aversion. The study is important at least for two reasons. First, it demonstrates that learning a link between an external stimulus and illness is possible and rather easy if the external stimulus is quite novel and salient. Secondly, these results are not in line with what one would expect from preparedness theory. If the organism is prepared for learning an association between taste and illness, it is hard to explain how this learning can easily be blocked by learning an artificial or unprepared contingency.

All these findings suggest that taste aversion is one particular instance of learning a relation between two events. However, it remains true that several characteristics of the Garcia findings were indeed exceptional. The importance of 'the message of Garcia' remains in the fact that it stimulated a new look at more conventional procedures. First the parametric differences, especially the time lag between CS and US, or between the discriminative stimulus and the reinforcer. The easiest explanation in terms of an after-taste was experimentally rejected (Revusky and Garcia, 1970). Taste aversion seems to be a central memory phenomenon: at the moment of illness the rat seems to remember the taste cue. Recent experiments by Lett (1973, 1974, 1975, 1977) have demonstrated that an analogous process can be demonstrated within more conventional procedures. Without going into the details of her experiments, it was shown that for learning the solution of a T-maze, a rat can bridge the interval between a choice response and the reward if—and only if—the situation is so constructed that the rat is 'reminded' of its choice response at the moment of reinforcement. It is rather remarkable that the Garcia effect, which is so deeply rooted in the biological condition of the living organism, has been a strong impetus to integrate recent theorizing on memory with conditioning phenomena. Next to this parametric difference, the Garcia effect was characterized by the interaction between cue and consequence. This interaction is only puzzling when one accepts extrinsic factors such as contiguity or contingency as necessary and sufficient. However, even within associationism, factors such as stimulus similarity, spatial coincidence, and others, have always been considered as of equal importance (Rescorla and Holland, 1976; Testa, 1974). The taste aversion paradigm was a strong incentive to study more carefully how these factors influence conditioning (Rescorla and Furrow, 1977; Rescorla and Cunningham, 1979). Finally, Garcia and others have always defended the position that there is a qualitative difference between taste aversion and other conditioning paradigms. According to this position, taste aversion reflects an hedonic shift: the taste is not bad inasmuch as it is a signal for eventual illness, but it becomes intrinsically a bad taste. This is a rather difficult question to answer (Gleitman, 1974). It might be related to the special characteristics within a taste–illness relation.

CONDITIONING AND ATTRIBUTION

In the first section, a brief survey was given of some studies demonstrating how an organism is sensitive to various aspects of information with regard to the relation of two events. In the second section, one particular form of inter-event learning was described: the taste aversion paradigm. Instead of postulating an innate mechanism, we are much more in favour of integrating these findings within the general study of inter-event learning (Revusky, 1977). From the preceding two sections, we would like to conclude that there is more than a superficial link between the conditioning literature and attribution theory. In other words, there seem to be common principles in the way infra-human and human organisms discover the causal network of their world. This rather speculative conclusion might warrant some preliminary remarks.

Attribution theory covers the study of how some events are explained by their eventual causes. Having been developed within social psychology, mainly by the seminal work of Fritz Heider (1958), the main event for which a causal explanation was studied was the behaviour of oneself or of another person. However, attribution theory essentially covers a much larger topic: how does an organism come to causal inferences for all kinds of events? It is even questionable whether a sharp distinction should be made between a causal analysis of events or occurrences 'things that happen', and the causal analysis of behaviour or action. This distinction goes back to the distinction between 'reason' and 'cause', which was the topic of a recent debate among social psychologists (Buss, 1978, 1979; Harvey and Tucker, 1979; Kruglanski, 1979). Within the context of this chapter, the distinction seems very helpful. We will only talk about causal inference of occurrences 'things that happen'. To put it rather trivially: if a rat receives a shock from the experimenter, it may ask a rudimentary question why the shock is given (a question about the cause), but not why the experimenter is giving the shock (a question about the reason). Both are 'why' questions, but logically different from each other. A second preliminary remark is related to the distinction between the process of attribution and the content of attribution. It is clear that, with regard to content, any comparison between humans and animals is meaningless; but even among humans such a comparison is difficult because of cultural differences (Kruglanski, 1979). However, with regard to the process of attribution, there might be some general epistemic rules which are common to humans and animals. Finally, a third preliminary remark is related to the concept of attribution itself. Attribution is conceived as a 'mediating concept' between input and output, but one can give it either merely an 'as if' character or a reality character. This is true for most mediating cognitive concepts. It seems to us that within social psychology, there is a trend to emphasize more the 'as if' character of attribution. In the original formulations, the sequence was schematically as follows: (1) something happens; (2) the organism asks 'why'; (3) it comes to a causal inference; (4) it reacts or behaves accordingly. Steps (2) and (3) are not observable. With humans, one can make them observable through verbal behaviour, and that is what most attribution research has been concerned with. Of course, at this level of research any comparison with animals is excluded. But there remains a central question with regard to the validity of these verbalized attributions. To illustrate this problem with Seligman's anecdote: when someone asked Seligman why he became sick, his answer would probably be 'because of the 'flu'. In other words, does any conscious reflection on the happening of an event obey different laws from the original global experience of the event? Is this not the truth behind the proverb of Pascal: *'Le coeur a des raisons, que la raison ne comprend pas.'* Nisbett and Wilson (1977) have recently made a strong argument that these cognitive mediating processes are not detectable by mere introspection. To validate their argument, they quote some cognitive psychologists such as Neisser and Mandler. Neisser writes: 'The constructive process (of encoding perceptual sensations) themselves never appear in consciousness, their products do' (Neisser, 1967, p. 301), and Mandler: 'There are many systems that cannot be brought into consciousness, and probably most systems that analyse the environment in the first place have that characteristic. In most of these cases, only the products of cognitive and mental activities are available to consciousness.' (Mandler, 1975, p. 245). Even while Nisbett and Wilson's argument may be partly criticized (Smith and Miller, 1978), several other authors are defending a similar thesis. Ellen Langer (1978) denies any mediating role of cognitions in most of our daily lives. 'Much psychological research relies on a theoretical model that depicts the individual as one who is cognitively aware most of the time, and who consciously, constantly, and systematically applies "rules" to incoming information about the environment in order to formulate interpretations and courses of actions. Attribution theorists rely on this model in attempting to uncover the sources of regularities in human behaviour. But if in fact it can be demonstrated that much complex human behaviour can and does occur without these assumed cognitive assessments, then we must question both the pervasiveness of attribution making as a cognitive process and the assumption made by most social psychologists' (Langer, 1978, p. 35). Similar arguments to formulate some simpler heuristics can be found in the writings of Kahnemann and Tversky (1973), Pryor and Kriss (1977) and especially Taylor and Fiske (1978). To mention only the conclusion of these last authors: '(Attribution processes) seem to occur automatically and substantially without awareness, and as such, they differ qualitatively from the intentional, conscious, controlled kind of search which we like to think characterizes all our behaviour' (Taylor and Fiske, 1978, p. 283). These preliminary remarks may give more credibility to the argument that there is something in common between men and animals in the way of inferring causal relationships between events.

To make a more direct link between conditioning and attribution, we would like to use the article of Kelley and Michela (1980) which summarizes ten years of attribution research. They start with presenting the general schema which is implicit in most attribution research (see Figure 3).

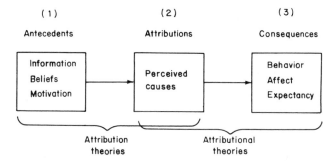

Figure 3. General model of the attribution field reproduced with permission from Kelley and Michela, *Annual Review of Psychology*, vol. 13, 1980

As was mentioned before, any direct study of (2) is excluded in animals. One is limited to a manipulation of (1) and from the observation of the output (3) one may infer what is going on in (2). But as was also argued before, this limitation by inference might also be true for the study of attributions in humans. If we now look more closely to the antecedents, there is a strong similarity, even an identity, with regard to factors influencing conditioning and attribution. Let us illustrate this similarity by mentioning some principles by which, according to Kelley and Michela, informational input is influencing the attributions. They are the same principles influencing conditioning (see first section of this paper).

Covariance

The ANOVA-model. This principle was introduced mainly by Kelley (1967, 1973). 'The effect is attributed to that condition which is present when the effect is present and which is absent when the effect is absent' (Kelley, 1967, p. 194). This principle is identical to the role of contingency within conditioning. According to Kelley, the principle of covariation goes back to a model of man being a naïve scientist constructing his causal network by means of the ANOVA-model. However, being influenced by covariation or contingency between events, does not imply any conscious notion of covariation or contingency and may reside in much simpler heuristics. There remains, however, a difficult question. How does one arrive from a contingency judgement to a causal judgement? A causal relation between two events implies contingency, but the opposite is not true. Is a causal judgement only possible if we know already from before the mechanisms by which cause and effect are related? Or are other factors, apart from contingency, necessary to perceive a causal relation. Is, in other words, causality a perceptual phenomenon or only a construction by reflection? (Michotte, 1954).

Saliency

'The notion here is that an effect is attributed to the cause that is most salient in the perceptual field at the time the effect is observed' (Kelley and Michela, 1980, p. 466). The role of 'saliency' in conditioning was already demonstrated by Pavlov (see above).

Similarity and contiguity

The role of contiguity in conditioning needs hardly any comments. Rescorla and Furrow (1977) have recently introduced some experimental procedures to study the role of neglected factors as stimulus similarity.

Primacy

'The general notion here is that a person scans and interprets a sequence of information until he attains an attribution from it and then disregards later information or assimilates it to his earlier impression' (Kelley and Michela, 1980, p. 467). One can discover the same principle within some findings of conditioning. When for instance a tone and a shock are randomly presented, but the series starts with some contingency between both events, the animal has some difficulty in discovering the randomness. The opposite seems also to be true: if one starts with a random series and then proceeds towards a contingency, the animal has trouble in finding out this contingency (Alloy and Seligman, 1979).

Next to these principles by which information leads to attribution, the role of previous 'beliefs' or causal schemata is evident within conditioning. 'Blocking' can be considered as a causal schema interfering with learning other causal relations: animals and humans seem to hold a sufficiency criterion with regard to causal explanations. Finally, the motivational component as an antecedent for attribution has always been central within conditioning: an animal seems only interested in the question 'why', when something important happens. Here, we are touching the main reason why we are talking of conditioning in terms of attribution. We prefer the term attribution instead of association, not only because association is an historically overloaded concept, but because it does not permit a distinction between the propositional knowledge 'event A reminds me of event B' and 'event A happens because of event B'. The behavioural consequences of both types of information may be quite different. To illustrate it again with Seligman's anecdote: at the moment of becoming sick, he can probably perfectly remember the whole dinner party, but he 'made an attribution' only with regard to the sauce béarnaise and he behaves accordingly. Memory is necessary but not sufficient to link two events in a causal network. 'Let us imagine that I emerge from my house in the morning and find a flat tyre on my car. It occurs to me immediately that around nine o'clock the previous evening, while driving home, I heard a disturbingly loud noise as I drove over something in the road. Now, 12 hours later, I "associate" the flat tyre with the impact. This is not an association in the usual S-R contiguity sense; rather, I have related two events which were separated by a long period of time. I can do this only if I have a record of the earlier event, or memory. In fact, I have many memories of previous events, *and that is the problem. The question to be dealt with is one of trace selection or contact, of how I have related these two particular events*' (Winograd, 1971, pp. 272–273, my italics). This quotation reminds us of the Garcia effect. As was noted by Revusky and Garcia: 'Probably, the rat can really associate these events (taste and shock) but will not attribute the production of shock to the flavoured water. In other words, a rat can learn that consumption of flavoured water *precedes* shock, but will not readily learn that consumption of flavoured water *produces* shock' (Revusky and Garcia, 1970, p. 41). And they conclude: 'This paper would probably be more precise if, whenever the term "association" is used, "attribution" were to be substituted' (Revusky and Garcia, 1970, p. 43).

CONCLUSION

Linking attribution theory and conditioning is not a purely academic exercise. It may have some consequences for the way we conceive various problems in a clinical context. In the past ten years, behaviour therapy has been 'going cognitive' and within this new look, it is even becoming old-fashioned to show any interest in such simple phenomena as conditioning. But just as in early attribution research, too much emphasis is given by cognitive therapists to conscious or semi-conscious private 'self-talks' of their clients. These self-talks are epiphenomena, 'surface structures', which might or might not be congruent with some deeper epistemic knowledge of their world. 'Unconsciousness' is a term to be avoided when discussing behaviour therapy. However, like taste aversion, this aversiveness might be totally irrational. The time has come to integrate current cognitive theories within our therapeutic endeavours. But in undertaking this challenge, we must not forget our roots: there is no place for dogma when we have to confess that we still do not know why Pavlov's dog was salivating when he heard the bell.

In conclusion, one could get the impression that within recent conditioning studies, one thinks of the rat as a small human being, whereas in earlier days one thought of a human being as a big rat. While respecting the specificity of each species, a total separation of both study domains is not very fruitful. In the introduction to the second volume on learning and cognition, Estes writes: 'The thought arises that the processes and mechanisms of human cognition represent specializations and elaborations of processes and mechanisms which can advantageously be studied in animals that learn as well as in machines that think' (Estes, 1975, p. 6). Estes' first alternative seems still worthwhile. As long as a computer does not salivate when he sees a piece of meat, we can still learn something from Pavlov's dog.

REFERENCES

Alloy, L. B., and Seligman, M. E. P. (1979) On the cognitive component of learned helplessness, in Bower, G. H. (ed.), *The psychology of learning and motivation*. Academic Press, New York, Vol. 13, pp. 219–276

Buss, A. R. (1978) Causes and reasons in attribution theory: A conceptual critique. *Journal of Personality and Social Psychology*, **36**, 1131—1321.

Buss, A. R. (1979) On the relationship between causes and reasons. *Journal of Personality and Social Psychology*, **37**, 1458–1461.

Estes, W. K. (1975) Introduction, in Estes, W. K. (ed.), *Handbook of learning and cognitive processes*. Erlbaum, Hillsdale, New Jersey, Vol. 2, pp. 1–6.

Garcia, J., and Koelling, R. A. (1966) Relation of cue to consequence in avoidance learning. *Psychonomic Science*, **4**, 123–124.

Gleitman, H. (1974) Getting animals to understand the experimenter's instructions. *Animal Learning and Behavior*, **2**, 1–5.

Harvey, J. H., and Tucker, J. A. (1979) On problems with the cause-reason distinction in attribution theory. *Journal of Personality and Social Psychology*, **37**, 1441–1446.

Heider, F. (1958) *The psychology of interpersonal relations*, Wiley, New York.

Kahneman, D., and Tversky, A. (1973) On the psychology of prediction. *Psychological Review*, **80**, 237–251.

Kamin, L. J. (1969) Predictability, surprise, attention and conditioning, in Campbell, B., and Church, R. (eds.), *Punishment and aversive behavior*, Appleton, New York, pp. 279–296.

Kelley, H. H. (1967) Attribution theory in social psychology, in Levine, D. (ed.), *Nebraska symposium on motivation*, University of Nebraska Press, Lincoln. Vol. 15, pp. 192–238.

Kelley, H. H. (1973) The processes of causal attribution. *American Psychologist*, **1973**, 107–127.

Kelley, H. H., and Michela, J. L. (1980) Attribution theory and research, in Rosenzweig, M. R. and Porter, L. W. (eds.), *Annual Review of Psychology* Annual Reviews Inc, Palo Alto, Vol. 13, pp. 457–501.

Kruglanski, A. W. (1979) Causal explanation, teleological explanation: On radical particularism in attribution theory. *Journal of Personality and Social Psychology*, **37**, 1447–1457.

Langer, E. J. (1978) Rethinking the role of thought in social interaction, in Harvey, J. N., Ickes, W. I., and Kidd, R. F. (eds.), *New directions in attribution research*. Erlbaum, Hillsdale, New Jersey, Vol. 2, pp. 35–58.

Lett, B. T. (1973) Delayed reward learning: disproof of the traditional theory. *Learning and Motivation*, **4**, 237–246.

Lett, B. T. (1974) Visual discrimination learning with a 1-minute delay of reward. *Learning and Motivation*, **5**, 174–181.

Lett, B. T. (1975) Long delay learning in the T-maze. *Learning and Motivation*, **6**, 80–90.

Lett, B. T. (1977) Long delay learning in the T-maze: Effects of reward given in the home cage. *Bulletin of the Psychonomic Society*, **10**, 211–214.

Logue, A. W. (1979) Taste aversion and the generality of the laws of learning. *Psychological Bulletin*, **86**, 276–296.

Lubow, R. E. (1973) Latent inhibition. *Psychological Bulletin*, **79**, 398–407.

Mackintosh, N. J. (1978) Cognitive or associative theories of conditioning: Implications of an analysis of blocking, in Hulse, S. H., Fowler, H., and Honig, W. K. (eds.), *Cognitive processes in animal behavior*, Erlbaum, Hillsdale, New Jersey, pp. 155–175.

Mandler, G. (1975) *Mind and emotion*. Wiley, New York.

Michotte, A. (1954) *La perception de la causalité*. Studia Psychologica, Louvain.

Neisser, U. (1961) *Cognitive psychology*. Appleton, New York.

Nisbett, R. E., and Wilson, T. D. (1977) Telling more than we can know: Verbal reports on mental processes. *Psychological Review*, **84**, 231–259.

Pryor, J. B., and Kriss, M. (1977) The cognitive dynamics of salience in the attribution process. *Journal of Personality and Social Psychology*, **35**, 49–55.

Randich, A., and Lolordo, V. M. (1979) Associative and nonassociative theories of the UCS pre-exposure phenomenon: Implications for Pavlovian conditioning. *Psychological Bulletin*, **86**, 523–548.

Rescorla, R. A. (1968) Probability of shock in the presence and absence of the CS in fear conditioning. *Journal of Comparative and Physiological Psychology*, **66**, 1–5.

Rescorla, R. A. (1969) Conditioned inhibition of fear, in Mackintosh, N. J., and Honig, W. K. (eds.), *Fundamental issues in associative learning*. Dalhousie University Press, Halifax, pp. 65–89.

Rescorla, R. A., and Cunningham, C. (1979) Spatial contiguity facilitates Pavlovian second-order conditioning. *Journal of Experimental Psychology: Animal Behavior Processes*, **5**, 152–161.

Rescorla, R. A., and Furrow, D. R. (1971) Stimulus similarity as a determinant of Pavlovian conditioning. *Journal of Experimental Psychology: Animal Behavior Processes*, **3**, 203–215.

Rescorla, R. A., and Holland, P. C. (1976) Some behavioral approaches to the study of learning, in Bennett, E., and Rozenzweig, M. R. (eds.), *Neural mechanisms of learning and memory*. M.I.T. Press, Cambridge, Mass., pp. 165–192.

Rescorla, R. A., and Wagner, A. R. (1972) A theory of Pavlovian conditioning: Variations in the effectiveness of reinforcement and nonreinforcement, in Black, A. H., and Prokasy, W. F. (eds.), *Classical conditioning*. Appleton, New York, (Vol. 2).

Revusky, S. (1977) The concurrent interference approach to delay learning, in Barker, L. M., Best, M. R., and Domjean, M. (eds.), *Learning mechanisms in food selection*. Baylor University Press, Waco, Texas.

Revusky, S., and Garcia, J. (1970) Learned associations over long delays, in Bower, G. H., and Spence, J. T. (eds.), *Psychology of learning and motivation: Advances in research and theory*. Academic Press, New York, pp. 1–84.

Rozin, P., and Kalat, J. W. (1972) Learning as a situation-specific adaptation, in Seligman, M. E. P., and Hager, J. L. (eds.), *Biological boundaries of learning*. Appleton, New York, pp. 66–96.

Rudy, J. W., Iwens, S. J., and Best, P. J. (1977) Pairing novel exteroceptive cues and illness reduces illness-induced taste aversions. *Journal of Experimental Psychology: Animal Behavior*, **3**, 14–25.

Seligman, M. E. P. (1970) On the generality of the laws of learning. *Psychological Review*, **77**, 406–418.

Seligman, M. E. P., and Hager, J. L. (eds.) (1972) *Biological boundaries of learning*, Appleton, New York.

Seligman, M. E. P., Maier, S. F., and Solomon, R. L. (1971) Unpredictable and uncontrollable aversive events, in Brush, F. R. (ed.), *Aversive conditioning and learning*, Academic Press, New York, pp. 347–400.

Smith, E. R., and Miller, F. D. (1978) Limits on perception of cognitive processes: A reply to Nisbett and Wilson. *Psychological Review*, **85**, 355–362.

Taylor, S. E., and Fiske, S. T. (1978) Salience, attention, and attribution: Top of the head phenomena, in Berkowitz, L. (ed.), *Advances in experimental social psychology*, Academic Press, New York, Vol. 11, pp. 250–288.

Testa, T. J. (1974) Causal relationships and the acquisition of avoidance responses. *Psychological Review*, **81**, 491–505.

Testa, T. J. (1975) Effects of similarity of location and temporal intensity pattern of conditioned and unconditioned stimuli on the acquisition of conditioned suppression in

rats. *Journal of Experimental Psychology: Animal Behavior Processes*, **104,** 114–121.
Winograd, E. (1971) Some issues relating animal memory to human memory, in Honig, W. K., and James, P. H. R. (eds.), *Animal memory*, Academic Press, New York.

Learning Theory Approaches to Psychiatry
Edited by John Boulougouris
© 1982 John Wiley & Sons Ltd

2. IS CONDITIONING RELEVANT TO BEHAVIOUR THERAPY?

Isaac Marks

Classical conditioning usually refers to the ways in which organisms come to associate events which are contiguous in time. More recently the importance of the similarity and spatial contiguity of events to be associated has also been recognized (see Chapter 1). This process has been extensively studied in animals and to a lesser extent in humans in laboratory experiments. The conditioning model has been widely used as an example for phobic and obsessive–compulsive disorders, the field which has been most extensively tilled by behavioural psychotherapists so far. It is important to examine how far this model can explain the phenomenology of phobias and rituals, including their acquisition and their reduction both naturally and in treatment.

There are at least four differences between aversive conditioning experiments carried out in the laboratory and their supposed clinical counterparts of phobias and rituals. First, the duration of the laboratory experiments is usually one day or a few days at most, whereas by the time they come for treatment phobias and rituals have generally been present for several years. Second, aversive conditioning experiments are generally one-off events, whereas human phobics and ritualizers commonly give a history of a stuttering start with repeated reacquisition and re-extinction of the problem before they become chronic and after which they can still fluctuate with many events. There is reason to believe that a single acquisition–extinction series may follow rather different rules from the same series repeated many times (Akiyama, 1968). Third, in laboratory conditioning experiments the initiating trauma is carefully planned and identifiable whereas with clinical phobics and ritualizers a history of an initiating trauma is usually absent and even vicarious conditioning is unusual (Rimm *et al.*, 1977). This suggests that for the majority of phobic–obsessive phenomena the initiating events, let alone the maintaining ones, may well be very different from those seen in a laboratory. This point is related to the next difference between the clinical phenomena and their experimental counterparts, namely that in aversive conditioning experiments the labels conditioned stimulus, unconditioned stimulus, conditioned response, unconditioned response (CS–US, CR–UR) are planned, identifiable, and have clear referents. In contrast, this terminology does not usually have clear referents in clinical situations. As an example, when an agoraphobic has anticipatory anxiety prior to going out alone, is this an internal conditioned response produced by an internal conditioned stimulus of going out, or is it the unconditioned stimulus or the unconditioned response? It could also be regarded as the conditioned stimulus. Thus the same clinical phenomenon could equally well be described by four very different labels, while in the laboratory each label refers to only one event. Clearly the laboratory terminology does not transfer easily to patients and an alternative language is desirable, of which more later.

A salient feature of phobias which cannot currently be explained by classical conditioning is the way in which childhood phobias wax and wane dramatically without obvious initiating trauma. This has been well-documented (Marks, 1969; Agras et al., 1971) in humans. An excellent experimental demonstration of this in rhesus monkeys was given by Sackett in 1966 in a neglected experiment. Rhesus infant monkeys were reared in total isolation from their peers. Every day over many months picture slides from four categories were projected on to one side of their cage. The frequency of the monkeys' disturbance to each category of slide was recorded, as well as the frequency with which the monkeys touched levers in order to obtain each of the four categories of slides. No disturbance was shown to any of the three categories of slides which showed other infants, other adult monkeys, or inanimate objects. The only category of slide to evoke disturbed behaviour was that depicting another monkey in a threat posture. The disturbance was first manifest at age two-and-a-half months, peaked at three months and waned sharply by four months, and had almost disappeared by seven months. Similarly, the monkeys increasingly touched levers which brought on a display of all four categories of slides but from age three months onwards the frequency with which they brought on those slides which depicted threat displays of another monkey dropped sharply and only rose again at four-and-a-half months, resuming the same level as other slides by age five-and-a-half months. It is also of passing interest that the monkeys worked less to obtain slides depicting neutral objects than slides showing monkeys in the three other categories (except for threat postures from age three to five-and-a-half months).

Sackett's experiment is perhaps the clearest experimental demonstration of the non-randomness of situations which evoke phobic responses and of the fact that at least some phobias are age-dependent. In humans fear of strangers tends to emerge most obviously between ages eight and twelve months, while fears of animals are most obvious from ages one-and-a-half to six years. In contrast wariness of heights is manifest in human infants as soon as they can crawl to avoid the 'visual cliff' in appropriate apparatus (Marks, 1969).

With respect to the waning of phobias in young humans, Agras et al. (1971) found in a five year follow-up of untreated phobics in the community that adult phobics largely retained their phobias when seen untreated five years later. In sharp contrast subjects younger than age 20 showed a marked reduction of their phobias almost to the point of extinction when seen untreated five years later.

This finding suggests that perhaps at least some of the explanation for the presence of phobias and rituals in adults is not their enhanced acquisition of these phenomena but rather their failed extinction (Marks, 1979; see Chapter 8). It is well known that almost everybody has marked fears at some time or another in childhood but most lose these phobias as rapidly as they develop them and very few remain phobic into adolescence and later (Marks, 1969). Anecdotally to a lesser extent this may also be true for obsessive–compulsive phenomena which seem to be a normal developmental phenomenon in many children roughly between ages five and eleven years, but this has not been studied systematically. The concept of failed extinction rather than enhanced acquisition as an explanation for the presence of some phobias and rituals is reminiscent of current immunological theories about the development of some cancers, e.g. breast cancer is very sensitive to changes in hormonal levels and perhaps to other immunological mechanisms. Tumour cells of certain kinds are commonly present in the organism but only in the absence of resistance are they able to take root and establish themselves. We are reminded here that in poor countries the tubercle bascillus has infected almost everybody but only a small proportion of the population develops active tuberculosis when infection is very heavy or resistance is lowered for a variety of reasons. The question of how we might enhance resistance to phobias and obsessions will be returned to later.

The non-randomness of situations which evoke phobias and rituals and the selective timing for the emergence of at least some of these has been explained by the related concepts of prepotency (Marks, 1969) and preparedness (Seligman, 1970). Prepotency indicates selective attention of the species (stimulus salience) to particular stimuli rather than others when these are encountered without previous experience. Preparedness indicates a selective facility to associate only certain stimuli with certain other responses, i.e. enhanced availability of certain S–R connections rather than others. One could perhaps think of greater and lesser S–R valencies in a manner reminiscent of chemical valencies. Another point is that the species has a readiness to make certain responses rather than others regardless of the stimuli leading to those responses. These ideas indicate that as a species we have been shaped to respond readily to certain stimuli of particular evolutionary significance, which may, of course, no longer be relevant to the changed situations of modern civilization, which has not been present long enough to materially alter man's genetic endowment.

An illustration of the difference between prepotency and preparedness comes from an anecdote by Lang. If one stares at a monkey it will show signs of arousal, being very attentive to eye contact (prepotency). However, it is less predictable if the arousal evoked by the stare will lead to any particular response, as the response may equally well be sexual presentation, escape or threat display. In contrast, preparedness would predict that a particular stimulus (being stared at) would evoke only one kind of response (perhaps threat in this instance).

An ingenious experimental paradigm attempting to demonstrate the phylogenetic proclivity of man to attend to fear relevant stimuli and to be resistant to extinction of responses to them was developed in Uppsala by Öhman (1978) and his collaborators in a 'differential conditioning' paradigm. In these experiments supposedly fear-relevant stimuli such as slides of snakes and spiders are presented repeatedly while paired with an unpleasant experience such as an electric shock or white noise. The effect on skin conductance, finger pulse volume, and heart rate is measured and compared with that of contrasting neutral slides such as paper tissues, flowers, and mushrooms. Only half the slides in each category are paired with an aversive US or unconditioned stimulus (CS$^+$ condition) while half are unpaired (CS$^-$ condition). Subsequent differences between the CS$^+$ and CS$^-$ slides indicate what conditioning has occurred, while discrepancies between the amount of differential conditioning shown to fear-relevant as opposed to neutral stimuli are an index of preparedness. In contrast, the initial orienting responses at the start of the experiment, before conditioning (paired) trials have begun, are an index of stimulus salience or prepotency.

Stimulus salience is often present in the data of workers using this paradigm. This is shown when initial responses to fear-relevant stimuli are larger than to neutral stimuli even before any pairing has occurred during the initial stage of habituation and at the very start of acquisition (pairing). This effect is not always present or significant. It is generally there for skin conductance data though not for finger pulse volume or heart rate (see Fredrikson et al., 1976; Öhman et al., 1976; Öhman, 1978; Fredrikson and Öhman, 1979; Hodes et al., 1981; Fredrikson, 1980). For heart rate salience is only occasionally present, e.g. before conditioning deceleration was more pronounced to potentially phobic than to neutral stimuli in the study of Fredrikson and Öhman, (1979), though heart rate did not subsequently discriminate between CS$^+$ and CS$^-$. It will be remembered that cardiac acceleration is the usual response to phobic stimuli in patients.

The presence of stimulus salience is unlikely to account for the differential 'conditioning' often found with this paradigm, or for the fact that a 'sensitization' group responds less to snake and spider slides than does a conditioning group (Fredrikson et al., 1976) for four reasons (M. Fredrikson and A. Öhman, personal communications). First, salience is not demonstrable for finger pulse volume even when this measure subsequently shows differential 'conditioning' i.e. phobic stimuli take longer than neutral stimuli to reach baseline during extinction. Second, differential conditioning between phobic and neutral stimuli was only found for an aversive US (shock) but not for a neutral US (tone), though stimulus salience was present initially for both US groups (Öhman, 1978). Third, complex stimuli (abstract paintings) did not condition more than did simple stimuli (colour only) despite the former having given larger preconditioning responses (Öhman et al., 1976). Fourth, salience is more obvious for dorsal than for palmar skin conductance responses, yet the reverse is true for differential 'conditioning' (Fredrickson, 1980). We can thus conclude that there is evidence for both prepotency and preparedness of fear-relevant stimuli, but that prepotency is not necessary for preparedness to occur.

Öhman and his coworkers have attended less to the stimulus salience often seen at the start of their experiments than to the difference between responses to the CS$^+$ and CS$^-$ slides when presented unpaired without the US in the last extinction phase of their experiments. After conditioning (acquisition, pairing) paired CS$^+$ fear-relevant slides commonly evoke more arousal than do CS⁻ slides, and this effect is greater than for neutral slides. The decrement slopes during extinction are usually parallel for CS⁺ and for CS⁻ slides. We will remember that the CS⁻ slides were never paired with a US, and so any decrease in response to them during the 'extinction' phase could be called 'habituation', while the same decrease to CS⁺ slides is called extinction because they earlier were paired with the US during acquisition. The fact that the 'habituation' slope to the CS⁻ slides and the 'extinction' slope to the CS⁺ slides are usually parallel suggests that habituation and extinction may reflect common processes of response decrement.

By the end of the ten to twelve extinction trials usually given by workers with this paradigm, the CS⁺ fear-relevant slides are still further from extinction than the CS⁻ slides, whereas the CS⁺ and CS⁻ neutral slides are usually comparable; this is usually regarded by the authors as evidence of slowed extinction to fear-relevant stimuli. It could be said, however, that because the decrement slopes in the 'extinction' phase are parallel for CS⁺ and CS⁻ slides, that extinction is not proceeding at a slower rate, but is merely taking longer to reach baseline because it commonly starts from a higher level at the start of the extinction phase.

Differential conditioning to unpleasant versus other facial expressions was reported in an experiment from Uppsala. Öhman and Dimberg (1978) found differential conditioning during extinction to angry faces compared with happy or neutral faces. To separate the possibility of cultural rather than phylogenetic preparedness underlying the differential conditioning phenomenon, phylogenetically old and phylogenetically new fear-relevant stimuli were compared in a thoughtful study by Hodes *et al.* (1981). They found that phylogenetically old fear-relevant stimuli such as snakes and spiders generated differential conditioning effects compared to neutral stimuli such as flowers and mushrooms, and compared to phylogenetically recent stimuli such as slides of rifles and revolvers pointing sideways away from the observer, which like neutral slides do not produce differential conditioning. One might argue that to be frightening the rifles and revolvers should point at the observer, not away from them, the latter presentation conceivably acting as a protective rather than a threatening stimulus.

With few exceptions the Öhman paradigm so far has not employed measures of the effects on subjective anxiety, and none have measured avoidance, both of which are critical variables. Moreover, the differential conditioning effect has only been demonstrated for skin conductance and finger pulse volume, not for heart rate (Fredrikson, 1980), whereas most phobics show tachycardia when in contact with their phobia-evoking stimuli. It has been suggested that this tachycardia of phobics developed as a result of their repeated experience of avoidance of phobic stimuli. This remains to be demonstrated.

The differential conditioning effect is rather fragile. While it has been repeatedly replicated in the original laboratory in Uppsala, attempts at replication elsewhere have met with variable success in Wisconsin, in Belgium (P. Lang and P. Eelen, personal communications), and even in a new laboratory of Öhman himself in

Bergen (A. Öhman, personal communication). Öhman pointed out that many subtle factors influence the differential conditioning phenomenon, only a few of which are recognized at present. One variable is the type of electrode used to record skin conductance activity from the finger. Eelen's laboratory used fluid electrodes, the finger being immersed in a cup containing saline solution, so that recordings probably reflected activity from both palmar and dorsal areas. This is potentially critical, as the differential conditioning effect is manifest more in the palmar area, which is thought to reflect sweat gland activity (Öhman, 1978) than in the dorsal area, which is said to reflect membranous reabsorption. Moreover, fluid electrodes lead to (1) hydrated swollen skin which occludes the sweat pores and so prevents sweat from reaching the skin surface and (2) activation of membranous reabsorption; fluid electrodes thus reflect activity of the membrane more than of the sweat gland, yet it is the latter which acts as an indicator of differential conditioning.

Another variable which might affect detection of differential conditioning is the nature of the US. The Wisconsin laboratory (Hodes et al., 1981) used a more aversive stimulus (loud noise) than the Uppsala laboratory (mild electric shock) and obtained much larger URs. This led to more conditioning of neutral stimuli, which by a ceiling effect might then have obscured any differential conditioning relative to fear-relevant stimuli. When in a later trial Wisconsin workers used a less aversive US of shorter duration than previously, the results more closely resembled those obtained from Uppsala, especially for instructed extinction.

Other differences are less well understood. Snakes behaved as fear-relevant stimuli both in Uppsala and in Bergen, whereas spiders seemed fear-relevant in Uppsala but neutral in Bergen, in the latter giving results like those from flowers and mushrooms.

The concepts of prepotency and preparedness concern the acquisition rather than the reduction of phobias and obsessions. Initially workers with the Öhman paradigm also found that in the extinction phase of their experiments instructions to subjects that the US would no longer be presented with the CS$^+$ immediately abolished responses during extinction to neutral but not to fear-relevant stimuli. However, Eelen found that this also abolished responses to fear-relevant stimuli (P. Eelen, personal communication). Furthermore, in the clinical setting presumably prepotent phobias such as spiders and snakes subside rapidly during exposure treatment. Inspection of the 'extinction' slopes in most Öhman-type experiments suggests that were more extinction trials given, in the way that they are during clinical treatment of phobias by exposure, that the response decrement would have soon declined to baseline levels.

The conditions governing this fascinating phenomenon thus need to be more clearly understood before it can be definitely stated that the paradigm marks the start of more sophisticated conditioning theory which can actually explain the non-randomness of situations which evoke phobias and rituals, and the selective ages at which many of these appear.

The Öhman paradigm is a significant methodological advance in that it opens up new ways of testing ideas about the manner in which new fears can start. The field would be even further enriched if workers extended it to include measures of subjective anxiety and of avoidance, ran longer series of extinction trials, ran repeated acquisition–extinction series in the same subjects, and took account of the ways in which the organism perceives the causal network of its world, as Eelen has suggested.

Another issue deserving more enquiry is the intriguing finding that differential conditioning, when present, is usually significant in the extinction phase rather than in the preceding acquisition phase. One wonders whether this points to incubation or other effects. It is worth examining the relationships between slope and magnitude of conditioning trials versus extinction trials, with special attention to relationships between the last conditioning trial and the first two extinction trials.

A phenomenological issue on which the conditioning paradigm has so far been silent is the differential association of various avoidance situations with the subjective and physiological events which occur when the subject is in contact with the relevant evoking stimuli. The first familiar association is that most phobic stimuli evoke fear, anxiety, and tachycardia. In contrast, another familiar combination is that blood–injury stimuli usually evoke a biphasic response consisting of initial tachycardia in the first few seconds after which nausea and a (presumably vasovagal) bradycardia becomes evident which can progress to cardiac asystole and fainting. These vasovagal phenomena are peculiar to blood–injury phobics, who usually have a history of repeated actual fainting after seeing blood (Connolly *et al.*, 1976), whereas actual fainting is exceptional in most other kinds of phobics despite a history of feelings of faintness, such as is common in agoraphobics.

Experiments remain to be done to demonstrate whether most non-phobic people also show (1) bradycardia to blood–injury stimuli after the first few seconds of contact, and (2) tachycardia to other types of phobic stimuli, but it does seem likely that this is a species response. How other species behave in this regard is not known. The phenomenon is reminiscent of death feigning in possums, and of the tonic immobility reaction in chickens and other species, a reaction which is indeed associated with bradycardia (Nash *et al.*, 1976).

A third pattern of association between one kind of avoidance reaction and its accompanying subjective experience is to be found in taste aversion. Taste aversion is associated with feelings of sickness or nausea, and the nausea seems different from the vasovagally induced nausea which is experienced by blood–injury phobics. Anxiety is not the usual experience associated with taste aversion, and the associated physiology is not known.

A fourth pattern of association is that found with sound and touch aversions such as those evoked by scraping chalk on a blackboard or feeling velvet. These aversions evoke neither anxiety nor nausea but instead are accompanied by shivers down the spine, and a feeling of the teeth being on edge (Price and Kasriel, 1972, reported by in Marks, 1978).

The fifth and final selective association of an avoidance behaviour with a particular subjective state is seen in many compulsive rituals. Rituals not uncommonly are associated with anxiety in the same manner as are phobias. However, situations which evoke rituals frequently also evoke not anxiety but rather disgust, distaste, or a sensation of uncleanness or stickiness. These associations remain to be mapped out systematically but if confirmed would need to be accommodated into any paradigm which is to be clinically useful.

Another phenomenological issue not yet handled by conditioning theories is the relationship between freezing responses and escape-avoidance responses during fear. In animals and in man the two response patterns can alternate but we do not yet know how to predict which will be evoked by a frightening stimulus. One might speculate whether the panic attacks seen in many agoraphobics and in generalized anxiety states are the internal equivalents of freezing reactions which in turn might be homologous to death-feigning or to tonic immobility reactions. It is also noteworthy that 'spontaneous' ('free floating') panic attacks not triggered off by an external or internal cue are common manifestations of anxiety states and agoraphobia, but rarely occur in other phobias and in obsessive–compulsive disorders. Why free floating panics occur selectively only with some anxiety syndromes and not with others is obscure but potentially important for aetiology and treatment.

Some differences between individuals in their readiness to acquire phobias and rituals are probably genetically based but how genetic differences are mediated to produce differences in fearfulness and in ritualizing is still a mystery. One could postulate that some physiological responses are normally distributed among individuals on a genetic basis, e.g. the thresholds for evoking vasovagal bradycardia and fainting to blood–injury stimuli. Those individuals with a genetically based extremely low threshold to this response are susceptible to blood–injury phobias. The same might apply to the triggering of height phobias, claustrophobia, and some agoraphobia; one could postulate that those with very low thresholds for evocation of the visual cliff phenomenon, or a sense of being confined or the discomfort of totally open spaces are liable, given sensitizing conditions like depression or increased general stress, to develop relevant phobias.

This brings us to the frequency of 'neurotic' types of depression in phobics and obsessive–compulsives (Marks *et al.*, 1980). In a substantial number depressive mood is associated with worsening of the fears and compulsions although in an unknown proportion phobias and obsessions actually improve as the depression worsens. The latter patients would naturally not present to a behavioural clinic. A conditioning model of behavioural treatment is so far unable to account for this association of pathologies. Ideas about learned helplessness do not explain it, as improvement in rituals and phobias does not lead to much improvement in mood at follow-up (Marks, 1971; Marks *et al.*, 1975).

Although conditioning models explain few features of the acquisition and phenomenology of phobias and compulsions, the reduction (extinction) of the psychopathology during behavioural treatment has some similarities to the process by which conditioned avoidance responses in animals can be diminished. The essence of both forms of behavioural treatment of phobias and rituals is to persuade the patient to come into contact with those stimuli which evoke distress and to remain in contact with those stimuli until the discomfort subsides.

The most efficient form of exposure is to bring the patient in touch with the real (*in vivo*) stimuli. Fantasied contact by imagining the evoking stimuli can also be therapeutic, but at a slower rate. Usually the reduction of discomfort takes up to several hours of exposure to be worthwhile, although there are notable exceptions where much briefer exposure has a rapid therapeutic effect. One could argue that once the patient learns that the discomfort subsides with continuing contact with the evoking stimuli and that there is no need to escape them or avoid them for improvement to occur, then the main therapeutic battle has been won. There is then no need for the patient to engage in phobic or compulsive behaviour in order to diminish the discomfort produced by initial contact with the relevant evoking stimuli.

Exposure treatments are usually effective in diminishing most phobias and rituals predictably and reliably and it can be given in many different ways. In a review the author (Marks, 1978) encountered 55 terms used to describe various forms of exposure. Exposure is an effective therapeutic tool whether it is given by psychologists, nurses, or doctors (Marks, 1981) and produces similar improvements whether given in Greece (Boulougouris, 1977), the USA (Foa and Goldstein, 1978), or Britain (Marks *et al.*, 1980). An important aspect of the exposure is that longer sessions such as two continuous hours of exposure has significantly greater effects than shorter sessions such as four half-hours with interruptions in between (Stern and Marks, 1973; Rabavilas *et al.*, 1976).

In laboratory experiments the 'flooding' experiments of Baum show important features in common with exposure treatments of clinical phobias and rituals. In Baum's experiments (1970) a rat was placed on an electrifiable grid at the base of a box. A few seconds later a shock was applied to the grid floor and the rat leapt about, soon discovering that a retractable platform was present half-way up one of the sides of the box, jumping on to it and thus being safe from further shocks. Within a few trials of being placed on the grid floor the rat soon learned to jump immediately on to the retractable platform before the shock was switched on. If now the shock apparatus was disconnected and the rat was again placed in the box it once more jumped immediately on to the platform, never learning that the shock had been switched off. The conditioned avoidance responses thus continued at this stage whether or not the grid floor was electrified.

If at this stage the platform is retracted so that the rat has no ledge on which to jump, then placing it on to the (now safe) grid floor leads to frantic attempts to jump on to a now non-existent platform which has been retracted. Within a few minutes the frantic jumping subsides and eventually the rat comes to remain quietly on the grid floor. As in the clinical setting, longer contact with the discomfort-evoking stimulus (the grid floor in this case) leads to more rapid decrease in avoidance responses. This form of extinguishing conditioned avoidance responses seems to be in the same stable as clinical treatments by exposure. Anything that leads to prolongation of 'functional CS exposure' (see Chapter 8) seems to hasten extinction, or perhaps one should say, reduction of the psychopathology.

It is not necessary to use the language of the conditioning laboratory to describe these events in the clinic. Instead of postulating unknowable unconditioned stimuli and responses one can simply speak about evoking stimuli and evoked responses that do not need the unlikely assumption that all cases have a history of traumatic or vicarious conditioning.

The response decrement seen during exposure treatments could equally well be termed adaptation, habituation, extinction, inhibition (conditioned, reciprocal, or external), exhaustion, 'gets used to it', or 'becomes bored with it'. The common element is response decrement. Some features of the different labels used for various kinds of response decrement are seen in Table 1. Among the relevant variables are the duration of contact with the evoking stimulus, the nature of that stimulus, and the nature of the response decrement involved. The table is merely a preliminary sketch of a framework within which to understand these phenomena in an integrated way.

Although exposure treatment is the most reliable way in which to obtain 'response decrement' with clinical phobias and obsessions, there are many examples in which improvement in phobias and rituals has been obtained by non-exposure methods. An obvious example is the value of antidepressants for reducing rituals in patients who already have depressed mood (Marks *et al.*, 1980), though how long the improvement would continue without any exposure is uncertain. Similarly, attempts to reduce fears by problem solving methods (see Chapter 7) or assertiveness training (see Chapter 11) also occasionally have some value. These effects are more fragile and less predictable than those of exposure. They do show, however, that at some point exposure treatment can be regarded as a kind of general coping treatment and that the teaching of coping skills may generalize towards the reduction of specific phobias and rituals.

The overlap between these differing approaches of coping and of exposure is only just beginning to be explored but could have far reaching implications. Knowledge about this area might tell us how far we can teach general stress–immunization to children in a long-term attempt at prevention of emergence of psychopathology, e.g. of generalized anxiety states. It has been documented that pre-exposure to situations such as dentistry, school, and separation from parents while in hospital can lead to reduction of fear in those situations. Such preventive work is potentially important and time will tell how specific we need to be to immunize against each type of psychopathology.

Meanwhile, it is clear that conditioning language is not especially useful to describe the acquisition and phenomenology of pathology, but there are interesting parallels between extinction processes in the laboratory and the reduction of psychopathology by the clinician. A common label could be 'response decrement'. Practising clinicians can largely disregard conditioning language and need terms

* Table 1. Labels for response decrement

Label	Duration of stimulation before phenomenon manifests	Recovery time	Nature of S	Nature of response decrement
Adaptation	Minutes	Minutes	US	Sensory receptor activity Central sensation
Habituation	Hours–weeks	Minutes–days	US	Any neuron or end target e.g. SC, HR
Extinction	Days–years	Days–years	CS	Any neuron, motor act, autonomic response (in absence of US)
Inhibition—reciprocal conditioned external		?	US/CS	
Satiation	Minutes–months	Hours–weeks	Pleasant/neutral US/CS	searching for or meaning of further S ? relates need to input
Exhaustion		?		
'Gets used to it'		?		
Boredom		?		

* Reprinted with permission from Marks, I. M. (1981). Cure and Care of Neuroses. John Wiley, New York.

more closely tied to the clinical phenomena which they are transforming. Concepts like state dependent learning might also need to be brought in to handle the fact that the mood state of the organism seems to affect the expressed pathology. We can expect future clinical paradigms to incorporate ideas from a variety of sources, including the conditioning laboratory, into a more sophisticated model better adapted to the clinical scene.

REFERENCES

Agras, W. S., Leitenberg, H., Barlow, D. H., Curtis, N., Edwards, J., and Wright, D. (1971) The role of relaxation in systematic desensitization. *Archives of General Psychiatry*, **25**, 511.

Akiyama, M. (1968) Effects of extinction techniques on avoidance response. *Bulletin of Faculty of Education, Hiroshima University*, **17**, 173.

Baum, M. (1970) Extinction of an avoidance response following response prevention (flooding). *Psychological Bulletin*, **74**, 276.

Boulougouris, J. C. (1977) Variables affecting the behaviour of obsessive compulsive patients treated by flooding, in Boulougouris, J. C, and Rabavilas, A. (eds.). *The Treatment of Phobic and Obsessive–Compulsive Disorders*. Pergamon Press, Oxford.

Connolly, J., Hallam, R. S., and Marks, I. M. (1976) Selective association of fainting with blood-injury phobias. *Behavior Therapy*, **7**, 8.

Foa, E. B., and Goldstein, A. (1978) Continuous exposure and complete response prevention treatment of obsessive–compulsive neurosis. *Behavior Therapy*, **9**, 821–829.

Fredrikson, M. (1980) Ph.D. dissertation, University of Uppsala. Unpublished.

Fredrikson, M., Hugdahl, K., and Öhman, A. (1976) Electrodermal conditioning to potentially phobic stimuli in male and female subjects. *Biological Psychology*, **4**, 305–314.

Fredrikson, M., and Ohman, A. (1979) Cardiovascular and electrodermal responses conditioned to fear-relevant stimuli. *Psychophysiology*, **16**, 1–7.

Hodes, R. L., Öhman, A., and Lang, P. J. (1981) Ontogenetic and phylogenetic fear-relevance of the CS in electrodermal and heart-rate conditioning (in preparation).

Marks, I. M., (1969) *Fears and Phobias*. Heinemann Medical/Academic Press, London.

Marks, I. M. (1971) Phobic disorders 4 years after treatment. *British Journal of Psychiatry*, **118**, 683–688.

Marks, I. M. (1978) *Living with Fear*. McGraw Hill, New York.

Marks, I. M., Hodgson, R., and Rachman, S. (1975) Treatment of chronic obsessive–compulsive neurosis by *in vivo* exposure. A two-year follow-up and issue in treatment. *British Journal of Psychiatry*, **127**, 349–364.

Marks, I. M. (1981) *Cure and Care of Neuroses*, John Wiley, New York.

Marks, I. M., Stern, R. S., Mawson, D., Cobb, J., and McDonald, R. (1980) Clomipramine and exposure for obsessive–compulsive rituals: I. *British Journal of Psychiatry*, **136**, 1–25.

Marks, I. M. (1979) Cure and care of neurosis. Salmon Lectures given to the New York Academy of Medicine, 30 Nov. 1978. I. Cure. II. Care. *Psychological Medicine* , **9**, 629–660.

Nash, R. F., Gallup, G. G., and Czech, D. A. (1976) Psychophysiological correlates of tonic immobility in the domestic chicken (gallus gallus). *Physiology and Behaviour*, **17**, 413–418.

Öhman, A. (1978) Fear-relevance, autonomic conditioning and phobias: a laboratory model, in Bates, S., Dockens, W. S., III, Gotestam, K. G., Melink, and Sjoden, P. O. (eds.). *Trends in Behavior Therapy*, Academic Press, New York.

Öhman, A., Fredrikson, M., Hugdahl, K., and Rimmo, P. A. (1976) Premise of equipotentiality in human classical conditioning: Conditioned electrodermal responses to potentially phobic stimuli. *Journal of Experimental Psychology*, **105**, 313–337, see pp. 320–1.

Öhman, A., and Dimberg, U. (1978) Facial expressions as conditioned stimuli for electrodermal responses: a case of 'preparedness'? *Journal of Personality and Social Psychology*, **36**, 1251–1258.

Price, J., and Kasriel, J. (1972) *Lecture to the Indian Psychiatric Society Silver Jubilee Meeting*, Chandigarh, India.

Rabavilas, A. D., Boulougouris, J. C., and Stefanis, C. (1976) Duration of flooding sessions in the treatment of obsessive–compulsive patients. *Behaviour Research and Therapy*, **14**, 349–355.

Rimm, D. C., Janda, L. H., Lancaster, D. W., Nahl, M., and Dittmar, K. (1977) An explanatory investigation of the origin and maintenance of phobias. *Behaviour Research and Therapy*, **15**, 231–238.

Sackett, G. P. (1966) Monkeys reared in isolation with pictures as visual input. Evidence for an innate relearning mechanism. *Science*, **154**, 1468–1472.

Seligman, M. (1970) On the generality of the laws of learning. *Psychological Review*, **77**, 406–1472.

Stern, R S., and Marks, I. M. (1973) A comparison of brief and prolonged flooding in agoraphobics. *Archives of General Psychiatry*, **28**, 210.

Learning Theory Approaches to Psychiatry
Edited by John Boulougouris
© 1982 John Wiley & Sons Ltd

3. THE RELATIONSHIP OF LEARNING THEORIES TO THE BEHAVIOURAL THERAPIES: PROBLEMS, PROSPECTS, AND PREFERENCES

G. Terence Wilson

'Once more unto the breach ...'

Ever since the emergence of behaviour therapy in the late 1950s as an alternative model of assessment and treatment to the prevailing psychodynamic approach, numerous discussions have focused upon the relationship between learning theory and the nature and clinical practice of behaviour therapy. The general thrust of these discussions, the arguments defending and insisting upon the fundamental relationship between learning theory and behaviour therapy (Eysenck, 1970; Wolpe, 1976) and the counter-arguments denying the existence let alone the desirability of such a relationship (Breger and McGaugh, 1966; Erwin, 1978; London, 1972), require little elaboration here. Rather, my purpose is three-fold. First, I wish to reaffirm the major contributions of classical and operant conditioning principles and procedures to clinical research and practice. Second, I want to restate the theoretical and clinical limitations of classical and operant conditioning approaches to human behaviour; they simply cannot serve as an adequate conceptual basis of behaviour therapy. Third, and most importantly, I wish to review alternative theoretical views that, building upon the hard won gains of behavioural research and therapy over the past 20 years, might advance our basic knowledge of psychological change and suggest innovative clinical treatment strategies.

THE IMPORTANCE OF BEING THEORETICAL

At the outset, I wish to reiterate the position that I have expressed elsewhere, namely, that theoretical developments have lagged behind in the general growth of behaviour therapy and that this does not bode well for the future of the field (Wilson, 1978b). In the period since Eysenck (1960) and Wolpe (1958) formulated behaviour therapy on the basis of what was then referred to *modern learning theory* (i.e. conditioning theory), the field has experienced remarkable growth. The two major advances have been the increase in technological know-how and versatility and methodological sophistication. New treatment techniques have proliferated and have been applied to an ever-expanding range of psychological, educational, and medical problems (Franks and Wilson, 1977, 1978, 1979; Kazdin and Wilson, 1978). The clinical practice of behaviour therapy continues to broaden and mature (Goldfried and Davison, 1976). Methodological refinements in the evaluation of the outcome of behavioural methods has occurred. A number of new applied research strategies have been developed (Hersen and Barlow, 1976), and the amount of clinical and more basic research within behaviour therapy continues to burgeon (Agras and Berkowitz, 1981). Behaviour research and therapy (including the pioneering journal itself!) are alive and well. Theoretical development, however, has failed to keep pace with this technological expansion and broadening applicability of behavioural methods.

W hy is a concern about theory important in contemporary behaviour therapy? Theory provides a means of integrating and interpreting available information and influences the search for new knowledge. Confronted with the increasingly apparent multiplicity of methods and concepts encompassed by the term 'behaviour therapy', a useful means of ordering the evidence, establishing priorities and filtering the good from the bad would be most useful. Whether viewed as loose metaphors or scientific theory, it is now widely accepted that the principles of classical and operant conditioning have been extremely successful in stimulating a wealth of experimental–clinical research and innovative therapeutic techniques over the past two decades. However, it can be argued that the heuristic value of these conditioning principles has peaked. Newer concepts (cognitive maps?) are needed to direct our research and guide clinical practice during the decade of the 1980s.

Scientific theory is also invaluable in making explicit the conceptual biases of a particular approach. Formulated so that its assumptions are testable and its procedures replicable, a theory makes it possible to refine, modify, or scrap pet therapeutic notions. Ideally, rival theoretical positions would be unnecessary if there were consensus on experimentally validated methods and outcomes. But this is a distant goal. In the meantime, unable to rely exclusively upon an empirically validated body of effective techniques, the therapist has to draw treatment strategies from some additional source. In short, the appeal is either to an organized conceptual framework or a melange of personal preference, intuition, and subjective judgment. Although the latter option will undoubtedly be helpful to some clients in certain situations, behaviour therapy has always been an attempt to improve upon this state of affairs by developing an applied science of clinical behaviour change.

Some applied behaviour analysts have characterized behaviour modification primarily as a methodological approach to personal and social problems. It is doubtful, however, that methodological criteria alone can define behaviour therapy or provide a basis for the choice of therapeutic strategies in clinical practice. One need only examine the theoretical differences between different approaches within the current compass of behaviour therapy. Although they share common methodological priorities and prize rigorous experimental evaluation of methods, applied behaviour analysis and social learning theory, for example, differ with respect to their conceptualizations of a model of human nature, causal processes in psychological functioning, and their implications for a technology of behaviour change (Bandura, 1977b, 1980; Catania, 1975; Goldiamond, 1976; Mahoney, 1974). The fact that theoretical issues and postures help to define behaviour therapy and influence basic and applied research is inescapable.

THE CONTRIBUTIONS OF CONDITIONING PRINCIPLES AND PROCEDURES

Ten years ago, I completed my doctoral dissertation on the extinction of fear and avoidance behaviour in rats. The findings, consistent with what was then known and has subsequently been reported, showed that avoidance behaviour was most effectively and efficiently eliminated by response prevention methods; conditioned fear was best extinguished through prolonged, continuous exposure to the conditioned fear stimulus (Wilson, 1973). It is of not inconsiderable significance that one can, with some confidence, assert today that *in vivo* exposure and response prevention methods, that derived directly from laboratory conditioning research, are the clearly preferred psychological methods for the treatment of phobic and obsessive–compulsive disorders (Boulougouris and Rabavilas, 1977; Marks, 1978; Rachman and Hodgson, 1980). This striking illustration of the value of contributions of conditioning principles to effective clinical practice is hardly an isolated instance. Among a variety of other successful extensions of conditioning concepts in the amelioration of diverse human problems, consider the many applications of operant conditioning procedures to childhood disorders, problems of classroom management, mental retardation, institutionalized psychotic patients, and so on (Kazdin, 1978; Leitenberg, 1976; Paul and Lentz, 1977; Ullmann and Krasner, 1975). The positive consequences of the application of conditioning principles and procedures to educational problems, psychiatric, and even medical disorders are now a matter of record.

It is often pointed out that procedures similar to those now employed routinely by behaviour therapists had been described well before the advent of behaviour therapy. However, the unearthing of historical precedents of procedures such as *in vivo* exposure, positive reinforcement, or even token economies is neither surprising (we would expect lawful and reliable influences on behaviour to have been noted by our more observant ancestors), nor in any way damaging to the view that the systematic application of conditioning principles to clinical disorders has greatly advanced our therapeutic effectiveness. The point that must not be overlooked is that specific behavioural procedures, whatever their heritage, were either ignored or rejected outright on highly debatable theoretical grounds by the dominant psychodynamic establishment in the 1950s and 1960s. The systematic use of direct behavioural methods in clinical practice is directly attributable to behaviour therapy. Moreover, the contribution of conditioning concepts went well beyond the introduction of particular treatment techniques. A more fundamental benefit was the conceptual and methodological emphasis that the study and application of conditioning principles brought to clinical research and practice. The detailed specification of therapeutic techniques, the focus on behaviour *per se* in assessment, treatment, and evaluation of therapy outcome, and the advances in measurement and methodology were all directly associated with the methodological behaviourism that characterized the conditioning approach.

This distinctive conceptual and methodological legacy of the influence of conditioning principles and procedures still serves to set behaviour therapy apart from alternative therapeutic approaches. Increasingly, it is argued that at least in different forms of brief psychotherapy, therapists, regardless of their theoretical orientation, are directive in their approach to patients and recommend behavioural practice (Butcher and Koss, 1978). Thus an attempt (*American Psychologist*, 1981) has been made to illustrate basic commonalities among diverse therapeutic approaches by arguing that most if not all approaches advocate corrective or extratherapeutic experiences. In support of this view, isolated statements by Freud, Fenichel, and other psychoanalytic authorities about the desirability of having patients try new ways of behaving in the extratherapeutic environment are cited. Gestalt therapy encounter groups and other approaches are similarly said to include an emphasis on specific behaviour change. Yet scholarly scanning of this sort of the vast literature on psychotherapy establishes only the most superficial commonality among diverse therapeutic approaches with respect to behavioural practice. It may be, for example, that psychodynamic therapists, particularly those who practise short-term treatment, do, on occasion, recommend some form of extratherapeutic experience outside of the therapeutic relationship, but this facet of psychodynamic approaches can hardly be likened seriously to the highly structured, explicitly scheduled, and systematically checked technique-specific and even problem-specific nature of *in vivo* homework assignments in behavioural assessment and therapy. The form and content of these various behavioural assignments in the client's natural environment have been heavily influenced by a reliance upon learning principles.

THE LIMITATIONS OF CONDITIONING THEORY

Classical conditioning

The classical conditioning model of the aetiology of phobias was pivotal in the early behaviour therapy formulations and treatment of neurotic reactions (Eysenck, 1960; Wolpe, 1958). Today, however, the inadequacies of a classical conditioning model of neurotic disorders are clearly apparent. Among the damaging lines of evidence are the failure of many people to develop phobias despite experiencing traumatic events, the absence of specific traumatic events in the life histories of most phobic individuals, the non-random nature of phobias, the lack of evidence that lasting conditioned fear reactions can be established in people under laboratory conditions, and the ease with which classically conditioned fear reactions extinguish in contrast to the often marked persistence of phobic disorders (Rachman, 1977).

Contemporary analyses of classical conditioning have moved away from the once popular notion that what was learned consisted of simple stimulus–response (S–R) bonds. In what is known as a molar account of classical conditioning, it is the learning of a correlational or contingent relationship between the CS and US that defines the conditioning process (Rachlin, 1976; Rescorla and Wagner, 1972). Classical conditioning is no longer seen as the simple pairing of a single CS with a single US on the basis of temporal contiguity. Instead, correlations between entire classes of stimulus events can be learned. This correlational view of conditioning more closely resembles complex behaviour than the simple one-to-one pairings of single CSs and USs that have traditionally been studied in classical conditioning experiments. The molar view provides an explanation for the first of the six problems with the conditioning model of fear reactions presented above. People may be exposed to traumatic events (contiguity) but not develop phobic reactions unless a correlational or contingent relationship is formed between the situation and the traumatic event. However, the molar view still fares poorly in accounting for the remaining problems with a conditioning model. It fails to explain neurotic fears where no traumatic event (US) can be identified, the selectivity of neurotic fears, or why neurotic fears, unlike classical conditioning reactions in the laboratory, are so resistant to extinction.

In sum, classical conditioning may be a factor in the acquisition of some fear reactions but cannot account fully for phobic disorders.

Mowrer's two-factor theory

Mowrer's (1960) two factor theory of avoidance behaviour, with its elegant yet robust simplicity, has been a fundamental building block in the development of effective treatment methods for phobic and obsessive–compulsive disorders. Despite its past utility, however, two-factor theory now encounters insurmountable problems in accounting for the experimental and clinical evidence on the maintenance and modification of neurotic disorders (Bandura, 1977a; Eysenck, 1981; Rachman, 1976). In brief, serious shortcomings include the difficulty in satisfactorily explaining the resistance to extinction of neurotic behaviour and the now well-documented fact that avoidance behaviour is not causally mediated by an underlying drive state of autonomic arousal (Herrnstein, 1969; Leitenberg, 1976; Rescorla and Solomon, 1967). There is no consistent relationship between autonomic arousal and avoidance behaviour. Avoidance behaviour often continues long after any classically conditioned anxiety (autonomic arousal) has been extinguished. Moreover, avoidance behaviour can be effectively eliminated without reducing conditioned anxiety. Anxiety reduction is sometimes the consequence rather than the cause of behavioural change and in both laboratory animals and clinical patients. A more accurate conceptualization is that both autonomic arousal and overt avoidance behaviour are correlated coeffects of some as yet undetermined central mediating state (Bandura, 1969).

Contemporary refinements of conditioning models of the maintenance and treatment of neurotic reactions do not overcome the various criticisms noted above.

Eysenck's revised theory of neurosis

The most serious attempt to improve upon the inadequacies of earlier classical conditioning and two-factor theories of neurotic behaviour is Eysenck's (1981) recent neo-behaviouristic S–R theory that bids fair to account not only for the aetiology, maintenance, and modification of phobic reactions, but also the more general phenomena associated with neurotic disorders such as spontaneous remission, the comparative outcome results of different therapeutic approaches, and even therapy-induced deterioration. A critical component of this revised theory is Eysenck's formulation of the incubation of fear hypothesis to explain the persistence of neurotic disorders under conditions that traditionally have been identified as necessary and sufficient grounds for extinction. In short, Eysenck argues that the basic law of extinction of a conditioned response has to be revised. In his view, presentation of an anxiety-eliciting conditioned stimulus without the unconditioned stimulus can result either in extinction of the conditioned response of anxiety (the usual effect) or the maintenance and enhancement of the conditioned response. The latter result is referred to as the *incubation effect*. According to this hypothesis, the conditioned response of anxiety has drive properties in the same way as the unconditioned response. Although Eysenck suggests some qualitative guidelines indicating when incubation as opposed to extinction might occur, the theory has little evidence to support it (Bersh, 1980). Moreover, it fails to account adequately for vicarious and symbolic influences in the acquisition and alteration of neurotic disorders (Wilson, 1978b).

Seligman's preparedness hypothesis

A number of investigators, including Eysenck in his revised theory of neurosis, have seized upon Seligman's (1971) suggestion that people are biologically prepared to learn certain fears as a result of our evolutionary past. This would explain the non-random distribution of fears and phobias people suffer from. Phobias about heights, germs, or snakes are more common than phobias about hammers or electric outlets because the former, and not the latter, were associated with danger and threats to life in our evolutionary history. According to Seligman, 'prepared' fears are often acquired on the basis of a single pairing with an aversive stimulus and are highly resistant to extinction. Laboratory studies of classical conditioning have shown that the specific nature of the CS can affect resistance to extinction. Hugdahl (1978) paired pictures of either snakes and spiders (a fear-relevant CS) or circles and triangles (the fear-irrelevant CS) with either electric shock or the threat of electric shock at the US. The dependent measure of CR was a change in skin conductance, a widely used measure of fear. All four groups of subjects showed equal evidence of conditioning. During extinction, when subjects were informed that no further shock would be given, the two groups who had been conditioned with the fear-irrelevant CS showed an immediate reduction in fear response. The two groups who had experienced the fear-relevant CS indicating resistance to extinction. Hygge and Ohman (1978) obtained similar results during extinction of a vicariously conditioned fear response. However, Seligman's 'preparedness' hypothesis is only one possible explanation of these results. An alternative view would emphasize differential social learning experiences. In our culture we learn to react quite differently to salient, fear-relevant stimuli, such as snakes, than we do to less salient stimuli such as circles and triangles. Other conceptual and empirical objections to the biological preparedness notion are presented by Bandura (1977b) and Delprato (1980).

Inconsistent with the notion of 'prepared' fears is the fact that contrary to the hypothesis, they do not appear to be unusually resistant to extinction in actual treatment studies. Phobias are readily extinguished in clients when the appropriate learning conditions are arranged. In a clinical test of the preparedness hypothesis, DeSilva *et al.* (1977) rated 69 phobic and 82 obsessional clients for the 'preparedness', or evolutionary significance, of their fears and related these measures to therapeutic outcome. The results showed that the 'preparedness' ratings failed to predict treatment outcome, stimulus generalization, severity of the problem, the suddenness of the onset of fear, or the age of onset.

The molar, correlational interpretation of avoidance behaviour

An interpretation of avoidance behaviour that is based on a correlational analysis of the relationship between behaviour and its consequences overcomes several of the objections to the two-factor theory of avoidance behaviour (Herrnstein, 1969; Rachlin, 1976). This correlational interpretation of avoidance behaviour is an operant analysis that assumes that avoidance behaviour is learned and maintained because it reduces or eliminates negative consequences. In contrast to two-factor theory, the concept of classically conditioned fear is said to be unnecessary. Avoidance behaviour is explained by analysing the observable relationship (correlation or contingency) between the organism's responses and environmental outcome, without any reference to an internal mediating state, such as fear.

The advantages of this operant analysis of avoidance behaviour are: (1) It is consistent with the evidence that clearly shows that fear is probably not a necessary condition for the learning of avoidance behaviour and is definitely not necessary for the maintenance of avoidance behaviour. Fear may affect avoidance behaviour, but it is not critical for its explanation. (2) This operant analysis leads to the prediction that the most efficient way of extinguishing avoidance behaviour would be to concentrate on the avoidance behaviour directly, rather than on the presumed underlying state of fear as in two-factor theory. This prediction is borne out by the clinical evidence. (3) Since a classically conditioned fear response is not the cause of avoidance behaviour in this analysis, it is easier to explain that resistance to extinction would take place only if the correlation between avoidance behaviour and outcome was broken. In order for this to happen, the organism must discriminate that the contingency has changed and that avoidance behaviour is no longer necessary to reduce or eliminate negative consequences; yet a major problem still remains. Phobic clients are not always successful in avoiding their feared situations or objects but retain their fearful avoidance behaviour. The correlational or contingent relationship between their behaviour and its consequences is broken (no objectively aversive event occurs), but extinction does not take place. The problem is that it is not the observable relationship between behaviour and its outcome that often maintains the neurotic reactions, but the client's *perception* or *cognitive appraisal* of that relationship.

APPLIED BEHAVIOUR ANALYSIS

The operant conditioning model of behaviour, upon which applied behaviour analysis is based, has the advantages of simplicity, parsimony, and theoretical consistency. It has been demonstrably successful in generating an effective (albeit relatively limited) technology of behaviour change and its recent extension to the field of behavioural medicine, among other areas, indicate that its force is by no means yet spent.[1] Nonetheless, there is a sense of conceptual staleness about applied behaviour analysis and a recognition that there is a tendency towards the repetitive application of known procedures to rather trivial matters—usually in the context of highly sophisticated methodology. This trend has been commented on by applied behaviour analysts themselves, who voice concern over the fact that applied behaviour analysis seems to be drifting towards applying behaviour analysis (Deitz, 1978). As Hayes *et al.* (1980) concluded after their analysis of the contents of the first ten volumes of *Journal of Applied Behaviour Analysis*: 'We are becoming less concerned with basic principles of behaviour, and more concerned with techniques *per se* ... The present data ... not only show that the old concepts are being increasingly ignored but also that no new concepts are emerging' (Hayes *et al.*, 1980, p. 283). Noting the dangers inherent in a purely technological approach, Hayes *et al.* (1980) call for a renewed emphasis on conceptual developments.[2] I would argue, however, that these innovative conceptual developments are unlikely to occur within the framework of the logic and assumptions of operant conditioning theory. Indeed, it can be argued that this framework, with its explicit eschewal of mediating constructs—cognitive or otherwise—is far too restrictive and restricting to look to as a source of fresh ideas and new perspectives for advancing clinical research and practice.

In the ultimate analysis, the criterion of utility or heuristic value must decide the relative merits of competing theoretical views in contemporary clinical psychology. Whereas classical and operant conditioning principles had what amounted to a revolutionary impact on the field in the 1950s and 1960s, operant conditioning accounts, increasingly, have had to rely upon *post hoc* analyses of more recent treatment methods and outcome (Wilson and O'Leary, 1980). For example, the well-documented efficacy of vicarious treatment methods, including covert, symbolic, and live modelling, were derived not from animal conditioning models but from social learning theory with its emphasis on cognitive mediating processes (Bandura, 1977b; Rosenthal and Zimmerman, 1978). The introduction of what are called cognitive behaviour therapy techniques, particularly the cognitive restructuring methods of Beck (1976) and Meichenbaum (1977), which show much promise in improving our therapeutic efficacy with a range of different problems (Foreyt and Rathjen, 1978; Rachman and Wilson, 1980), derived directly from a cognitive mediational model of behaviour. Even if it were to be conceded that these methods could be accommodated within the *post hoc* parsimony of a non-mediational operant conditioning framework—a Procrustean manoeuvre not without controversy—the failure of the latter to generate such techniques is the telling point.

The foregoing has faulted the operant conditioning approach on the basis of what I submit is its faltering heuristic value. This non-mediational model has also been criticized as inadequate for conceptualizing such important psychological functions as self-regulatory and cognitive processes that are central to behaviour change (Bandura, 1977b; Bower, 1978; Erwin, 1978; Mahoney, 1974).

Finally, attention must be drawn to the fact that the traditional conditioning formulations of behaviour therapy have fallen far short of providing an adequate conceptualization of interpersonal influences in the assessment and modification of behaviour. This deficit is all the more important now that behaviour therapists appear increasingly to involve the client's spouse or family members in the over-all treatment process, examples of which include the treatment of alcoholism, agoraphobia, and obesity, and because of the recent developments in behavioural marital therapy. In this connection, the recent spirited interchange between Jacobson and Weiss (1978) who have spelled out the merits of a behavioural conceptualization of marital conflict and its treatment, on the one hand, and Gurman and his colleagues (Knudson *et al.* 1979) who, on the other hand, have criticized what they take to be the conceptual shortcomings of a strictly behavioural formulation, makes for instructive reading. The behavioural approach to marital therapy is based upon the assumption that reciprocity of positive exchange is the core characteristic of a successful marriage. This conceptualization is really an extension of Thibaut and Kelly's (1959) social exchange theory that holds that individuals are mutually striving to maximize rewards while minimizing costs. Suffice it to say that at a conceptual level, the rudimentary analysis of marital relationships in terms of simple reciprocal exchanges of positive reinforcement of desired behaviour fails to do justice to the complexity of dyadic relationships.

Contemporary behavioural treatment techniques for marital conflict have a mixed pedigree, deriving variously from the operant conditioning model, cognitive restructuring concepts, and even communication analyses of interpersonal interactions (O'Leary and Turkewitz, 1978; Weiss, 1979). The reliance upon communication analyses of interpersonal behaviour cannot readily be incorporated within the operant conditioning model of either the nature of dysfunctional relationships or the nature of effective change mechanisms as Knudson *et al.* (1979) are quick to point out. Yet the initial evidence strongly suggests that the communication training component of behavioural marital therapy is probably essential for effective treatment. As Jacobson himself has noted: 'It may be that the most effective element in the behavioural approach (to the treatment of marital problems, i.e. communication training) is the one which is the least unique to the behavioural approach' (Jacobson, 1978, p. 425). In short, behavioural marital therapy is a technology in search of an integrative theoretical framework—a conclusion that seems largely applicable to clinical behaviour therapy as a whole.

ALTERNATIVE THEORETICAL FRAMEWORKS

There simply is not a single, integrative theory that encompasses the diverse methods and applications of the different behaviour therapies. However, there are theoretical frameworks, in step with if not derived directly from developments in scientific psychology, that are preferable to conditioning concepts on several grounds and that show distinct promise of advancing our knowledge of behaviour change mechanisms and methods.

The broadest and in many ways the most sophisticated conceptualization of the behaviour therapies in Bandura's (1969, 1977b) social learning theory.[3] In his classic 1969 text, *Principles of Behavior Modification*, Bandura asserted that behaviour is developed, maintained, and modified on the basis of three distinct regulatory systems, comprising (1) external antecedent events; (2) the situational consequences of behaviour; and (3) cognitive mediating processes, including vicarious learning, symbolic activities, and self-control functions. To quote Bandura: 'At this higher level stimulus inputs are coded and organized; tentative hypotheses about the principles governing the occurrence of rewards and punishments are developed and tested on the basis of differential consequences accompanying the corresponding actions; and, once established, implicit rules and strategies serve to guide appropriate performances in specified situations. Symbolically generated affective arousal and covert self-reinforcing operations may also figure prominently in the regulation of overt responsiveness.' (Bandura, 1969, p. 63.)

Bandura (1969) claimed that these cognitive mediating processes were the most influential regulatory system, a position that committed social learning theory to explanatory constructs more in line with cognitive than conditioning theory. Throughout the 1970s social learning theory has increasingly reflected the influence of contemporary developments in information processing and other areas of cognitive psychology. In the course of this evolution, social learning theory, as Rosenthal points out, 'has made fairly intimate contact with research—mainly published in non-applied journals—that seems to have had less impact on most other neobehavioural and cognitively-oriented clinical standpoints ... From the font of basic research has sprung social learning theory's frame-of-reference. It attempts more articulation of component mental processes than would seem defensible if the burgeoning experimental literature were not addressed. Those studies collectively argue for a conception of symbolic activity along the lines adopted by social learning theory'. (Rosenthal, 1981, p. 00).

I have detailed my views about the merits of social learning theory as a conceptual framework for the behaviour therapies elsewhere (Wilson, 1978a; Wilson and O'Leary, 1980). To summarize, it can be argued that it provides a more comprehensive and integrative account of the facts of behaviour change than competing theoretical frameworks; it is testable; and it is heuristic in that it continues to spur and direct basic and clinical research and therapeutic applications. While the reader is referred to other discussions of these points, there is one aspect of this approach that I wish to elaborate upon here. Central to the evaluation of the adequacy of social learning theory is its commitment to explanation based on cognitive constructs, and it is to this critical issue that I now turn.

The cognitive connection

I submit that no theoretical account of the behaviour therapies can be successful without an adequate analysis of the role of cognitive mediational processes in the regulation of behaviour. It is a basic assumption of social learning theory and the other frameworks outlined in this brief survey of alternative conceptualizations of the behaviour therapies that the influence of environmental events on the acquisition, maintenance, and modification of behaviour is heavily determined by cognitive processes. These cognitive processes are based upon prior experience and govern what environmental events are attended to, how they are perceived and processed, whether or not they will be remembered, and how they might affect future thought and action. More recently, Bandura (1980) has also emphasized that the importance of cognitive processes is not limited to the encoding of immediate environmental stimuli, but also involve deliberate and self-referent thought that influences behaviour.

A focus on cognitive mediation is eschewed by operant conditioners. The influence of current cognitions is subsumed under the accommodating rubric of the person's 'past history of reinforcement'. Instead of talking about the processing of environmental information, the operant conditioner externalizes the explanation by suggesting that the person is reacting not only to the present environment, but also to past learning. Rachlin summarizes this viewpoint in stating: 'Inferences about past experiences may be as speculative about present cognitions, but at least they are potentially observable and suggest methods of observation and modification short of brain surgery' (Rachlin, 1977, p. 374).

Three important points must be noted in this connection. The first is that this dependence on a person's past history of reinforcement is inconsistent with the clinical practice of behaviour therapy, a cardinal principle of which is the emphasis on the variables that are currently maintaining the client's problems. The second point is that radical behaviouristic explanation, as Rachlin (1977) makes clear, necessarily involves an inference. Radical behaviourism is not free from inferential reasoning, as is commonly supposed. The question is not whether inferences will be made in trying to account for human behaviour, but what sort of inference is the most useful. This is an empirical question that will be decided ultimately by appropriate research, rather than by theoretical arguments. The third point is that the radical behaviourist is betting that inferences that do not involve cognitive variables will lead to more effective treatment methods than those that do. This latter position can be seriously questioned as I indicate throughout this chapter.

In contrast to a strict operant conditioning approach, neo-behaviouristic S–R theorists such as Eysenck (1981) and Wolpe (1958, 1976) have always explicitly held to a mediational model of behaviour, although the mediational mechanisms, however, have been non-cognitive (e.g. Mowrer's two-factor theory of avoidance behaviour). Cognitive factors in clinical practice have received very limited attention. Symbolic processes such as imagery were conceptualized within a covert conditioning model. Although heuristic and a useful historical link between radical behaviourism and more recent cognitive-behavioural approaches, the covert conditioning model is inadequate for the task of integrating cognitive mediating processes within a behavioural framework (Mahoney, 1974). Predictably, the current emphasis on cognitive processes in behaviour therapy has come in for strong criticism (Eysenck, 1979; Wolpe, 1976). It is important to point out that these attempts to undo the cognitive connection in behaviour therapy follow directly from a more fundamental objection to cognitive psychology in general. Never one to equivocate, Eysenck asserts that cognitive psychology is characterized by: 'an uncritical, or selective, or frankly cavalier attitude to experimental data; a pervasive atmosphere of special pleading; a curious parochialism in acknowledging even the existence of other workers, and other approaches, to the phenomena under discussion; interpretation of data relying on multiple, arbitrary choice-points; and underlying all else, the near vacuum of theoretical structure within which to inter-relate different sets of experimental results, or to direct the search for significant new phenomena.' (Eysenck, 1979, p. 513).

A different appraisal of cognitive psychology and its relationship to the behaviour therapies is typified in the following statement by Bower: 'It seems to me that social learning theory is a form of cognitive psychology that is being applied ingeniously to issues of socialization, of personality development, psychopathology, and behaviour modification. I think it is time for people to see that behaviour modification technology could just as well rest on cognitive psychology as on S–R conditioning theory. Certainly in comparison to S–R conditioning theory, cognitive psychology provides a more facile account of many recent therapeutic techniques such as covert modeling, thought control, self-instructional training, cognitive restructuring, persuasion, and—as Brewer (1974) argues—perhaps even the more direct operant conditioning procedures themselves. Since social learning theory and cognitive psychology seem to have been sleeping together for years, I think it is high time that we announce their up-coming wedding.' (Bower, 1978, pp. 145–146).

Acknowledging the necessity of paying serious attention to cognitive processes in behaviour change would seem to be keeping pace with developments in psychology that have taken us beyond the more narrow and earlier stage when conditioning theory dominated the experimental scene. Whether or not this recent emphasis on cognitive concepts will significantly improve our understanding and treatment of emotional disorders remains to be seen. We shall never know unless we try. Critics who seem certain that a cognitive viewpoint is misguided, or worse, likely to bring disrepute to the behaviour therapies, seem oddly out of tune with the spirit that helped give rise to behaviour therapy in the first place. After all, it is an approach to clinical research and practice that for the most part has been marked by bold and imaginative innovations, a vigorous diversity of viewpoints, and a healthy appeal to empirical data rather than authority figures or conventional thinking as the final arbiter of theoretical disputes.

Note that an emphasis on the importance of cognitive processes in the behaviour therapies does not necessarily mean acceptance of cognitive treatment methods or the specific assumptions on which they are based.[4] In terms of social learning theory, for example, the most effective treatment procedures are considered to be those that rely upon direct behavioural intervention, even though cognitive mechanisms are invoked to explain their effects. This distinction between *procedure* and *process* in clinical practice is often obscured in the literature of what has come to be called cognitive behaviour therapy (Wilson and O'Leary, 1980). Indeed, one of the major deficits of cognitive behaviour therapy is the lack of a satisfactory theoretical framework (Mahoney and Arnkoff, 1978; Meichenbaum and Cameron, 1981). The loose assumptions on which Ellis' (1977) rational-emotive therapy (RET) rests fall far short of a formal theoretical model. Moreover, their validity is very questionable (Craighead *et al.*, 1979). Beck's (1976) cognitive therapy and Meichenbaum's (1977) self-instructional training contain several important propositions about specific psychological disorders and their modification, but neither constitutes a comprehensive view of behaviour change mechanisms or methods comparable to that of social learning theory.

Self-efficacy theory

As Rosenthal (1981) points out, social learning theory is a general conceptual approach that encompasses a number of more narrowly-focused or relatively specific mini-theories. Examples include explanations of vicarious learning (Rosenthal and Bandura, 1978), self-control (Bandura, 1976, 1980), self-referent processes (Bandura, 1980), and the role of perceived competence (self-efficacy) in behavioural change

(Bandura, 1977a). Self-efficacy theory is of particular interest in the present context since it offers an alternative explanation of the action of commonly used treatment procedures such as systematic desensitization and flooding that have long been associated with classical conditioning concepts and two-factor theory formulations of behaviour therapy.

According to Bandura (1977a), treatment techniques such as desensitization, flooding, and variants of modelling are effective because they increase the client's expectations of personal efficacy. Efficacy expectations reflect a subjective estimate that one has the where-with-all to cope successfully with threatening situations. They are differentiated from outcome expectations which are defined as the client's belief that particular actions will result in certain outcomes. This mini-theory specifies the sources of information from which efficacy expectations derive and the major sources through which different modes of treatment operate. As Bandura (1980) observes, this line of reasoning overlaps with alternative cognitive–behavioural perspectives on the fundamental phenomenon of an individual's sense of perceived control over his or her life (Perlmuter and Monty, 1980).

Self-efficacy theory has aroused controversy within the field of behaviour therapy as documented by the conflicting evaluations of its value in Rachman's (1978) comprehensive anthology on the subject. My own view is that this is the sort of theory that makes an important contribution to the continuing growth of the behaviour therapies. As an explanation of the maintenance and modification of phobic disorders in particular, self-efficacy theory must contend with the problems encountered by conditioning theories in this regard. In fact, several of the problems noted in regard to the classical conditioning and two-factor theories are more easily understood in terms of this social learning perspective. In the discussion of two-factor theory it was pointed out that autonomic arousal does not directly motivate avoidance behaviour. Autonomic arousal and avoidance behaviour are correlated coeffects which, according to self-efficacy theory, are both products of expectations of personal harm or threat.

Can the theory account for the persistence of phobic disorders? The view is that the threat of personal vulnerability, acquired on the basis of any of the different sources of efficacy information, is maintained because the phobic selectively attends to and perceives cues and consequences, however improbable, that generate a sense of inability to cope. The exposure phobics have to their feared situations or objects, and which should produce extinction of conditioned anxiety responses, does not automatically alter fearful expectations. Whether these fearful expectations are disconfirmed and phobic behaviour hence eliminated will depend on the nature of the information the person derives from exposure with the phobic situation. If the exposure to the phobic situation is such that the person concludes that he or she can cope effectively with the situation without experiencing undue anxiety, then extinction will progress rapidly. If the exposure is such that the person concludes that he or she cannot cope and will experience unnerving anxiety, no extinction will take place. By strengthening the person's expectation that he or she cannot cope, the exposure might enhance phobic sensitivity.

Behavioural treatment methods for fear reduction, particularly techniques such as *in vivo* exposure or participant modelling, are demonstrably effective in overcoming phobic and obsessive–compulsive disorders in a majority of cases (Marks, 1978; Rachman and Hodgson, 1980). What we still do not understand is how these different techniques produce therapeutic improvement. Earlier conditioning explanations are simply unequal to the task. Among the findings that undermine these theories are: (1) the absence of the firmly predicted relationship between level of anxiety during exposure and treatment outcome; (2) the variability in treatment outcome under similar conditions of exposure; and (3) the evidence that the objective condition of exposure to the feared situation alone is insufficient for obtaining improvement. An important consideration is what it is that the person does during exposure and how he or she perceives the feared situation. Self-efficacy theory would seem able to account for these various findings (Wilson and O'Leary, 1980), but until the necessary experiments are completed, this must remain conjecture.

What is the current evidence on self-efficacy theory? Initial studies with snake phobic subjects by Bandura and his associates have shown that efficacy expectations accurately predicted reductions in avoidance behaviour irrespective of whether they were created by participant modelling, symbolic modelling, covert modelling, or systematic desensitization (Bandura, 1977a; Bandura *et al.*, 1980). Moreover, measures of personal efficacy predicted differences in coping behaviour by different individuals receiving the same treatment, and even specific performances by subjects in different tasks. Consistent with the theory, participant modelling, a performance-based treatment, produced greater increases in level and strength of efficacy expectations and in related behaviour change. Nor do these favourable findings appear limited to the optimal conditions of experimental control that the laboratory treatment of snake phobias provides. Demonstration of close congruence between efficacy expectations and improvements in coping behaviour at the level of specific tasks by agoraphobics (Bandura *et al.*, 1980; Williams and Rappoport, 1980), clients with simple phobias (Biran and Wilson, 1980), and psychiatric in-patients with heterosocial anxiety (Barrios, 1979) indicate that the theory has generality across different areas of functioning. Biran and Wilson (1980) found that congruence between self-efficacy and behavioural outcome in clients treated with cognitive restructuring was less than that achieved with the techniques mentioned above, but none the less substantial. In his studies with snake-phobic subjects, Bandura has consistently found significant correlations between efficacy expectations and self-reported fear arousal. This congruence, Bandura suggests, provides support for his social learning analysis of fear arousal in terms of perceived inefficacy or vulnerability. However, Bandura *et al.* (1980) do not report a similar finding in their study with agoraphobics, while Biran and Wilson (1980) failed to find a significant correlation between efficacy expectations and either self-reports or physiological measures of fear arousal. Neither did Barrios (1979) obtain this predicted relationship in his participant modelling treatment. These mixed results call for more detailed analyses of the hypothesized relationship between self-efficacy and fear arousal across different techniques and disorders.

The issue of generalization and maintenance of treatment-produced change loom large in contemporary research and practice in the behaviour therapies and they pose major problems for any theoretical analysis (Franks and Wilson, 1978). According to Bandura's theory, the level, strength, and generality of efficacy expectations should determine generalization of behaviour change. Encouragingly, the initial data suggest that perceived efficacy might be a better predictor of avoidance behaviour on measures of generalization in unfamiliar tasks than actual behaviour in the treatment setting.

Efficacy expectations must be predicted to affect maintenance of therapeutic improvement since the theory makes the assumption that they influence the amount of effort that will be expected to maintain coping behaviour, and the length of time this behaviour will be sustained despite adverse pyschological experiences. One month follow-ups of snake-phobic subjects treated with participant modelling have been consistent with this prediction (Bandura, 1977a). However, Barrios' (1979) data are inconsistent with the theory. He found that the number of coping responses patients made when confronted with aversive stimulation was unrelated to the strength of efficacy expectations.

A searching test of the predictive power of self-efficacy theory with respect to the maintenance of behaviour change is provided by studies on the treatment of addictive disorders. These disorders are notorious for their high relapse rates and adequate predictors of long-term therapeutic success and have proved to be uncommonly elusive (Miller, 1981; Wilson and Brownell, 1980). Studies by DiClemente (1981) and Condiotti and Lichtenstein (1980) on the treatment of cigarette smoking have yielded impressive support for self-efficacy theory. In the latter investigation, for example, efficacy expectations predicted both which subjects would relapse and how long they remained abstinent before relapsing at a statistically significant level. Even more instructive is the fact that there was remarkably high congruence between the situations about which clients reported low efficacy expectations and the nature of the situation in which they first resumed smoking ($k_w = 0.89$). Yet in a closely related study, Cooney (1980) failed to find the predicted relationship between self-efficacy and smoking rates at a three or six month

page 49

In the treatment of obesity, Collins (1980) obtained no relationship between measures of efficacy expectations of coping with high risk situations for uncontrolled eating and maintenance of weight loss during a one-year follow-up. It is doubtful, however, whether this represents a fair test of self-efficacy theory. It would make better sense to relate efficacy expectations to occurrences of uncontrolled eating episodes than to weight loss *per se*. Self-efficacy theory predicts behaviour change, and we know that alterations in eating habits do not necessarily result in consistent weight loss (Wooley *et al.*, 1979). The concept of self-efficacy has been incorporated in a comprehensive cognitive-behavioural analysis of the prevention of relapse in addictive disorders by Marlatt and Gordon (1979). In a test of this model of relapse with obese individuals, Rosenthal and Marx (1979) obtained confirmatory results. Regardless of the ultimate fate of specific self-efficacy theory, cognitive-behavioural analyses of the maintenance of behaviour change along the lines suggested by Marlatt and Gordon (1979), Rodin (1978), and Wilson (1978a) appear to bear importantly on the therapeutic challenge of facilitating lasting treatment-produced change.

Learned helplessness theory

Another theory of behavioural and emotional disorders that is based on the cognitive construct of *expectations* is Seligman's (1975) notion of learned helplessness. According to this theory, a person who is subjected to uncontrollable aversive consequences learns that his or her responses are futile and comes to expect that future responding will be similarly futile. This expectation, or learned helplessness, can result in severe emotional and motivational effects, including stress, adverse physiological consequences, and extreme passivity or the failure to initiate coping responses even when behavioural consequences are controllable. A revised version of the theory incorporates an emphasis on attributional processes in producing learned helplessness (Abramson *et al.*, 1978). Attributions of responsibility for helplessness to a lack of personal competence are said to be necessary mediators of the chronicity and generality of depression. This reformulation of the theory makes it difficult to distinguish Seligman's theory from self-efficacy theory (Bandura, 1978).

   In contrast to the broad implications of self-efficacy theory, Seligman's learned helplessness theory has been limited to the analysis of depression. Moreover, despite the sudden explosion of research on cognitive mechanisms in depression that it has sparked, learned helplessness theory, unlike social learning theory, has not had a noticeable influence on therapeutic practice. The treatment methods that the theory would suggest are in fact those that Beck (1976) had previously described in his well-known cognitive therapy for depression—directive therapy aimed at prompting the client to initiate behaviour that results in success experiences (personal efficacy) and which serve to dispel negative attitudes about the self and the environment. The therapy outcome data, such as they are, strongly indicate that cognitive-behavioural treatment strategies such as those developed by Beck are effective in treating some forms of depression (McLean and Hakstian, 1979; Rush *et al.*, 1977). These findings attest further to the necessity of broadening the behaviour therapies to take account of cognitive processes and procedures.

EMOTIONAL PROCESSING

If the behaviour therapies must take serious account of cognitive factors, they cannot afford to do this at the expense of de-emphasizing emotional or affective processes in psychological dysfunction. Contemporary cognitive psychology, as Zajonc (1980) has documented, simply ignores emotion. In a related vein, Mahoney (1980) has constructively criticized current cognitive behaviour therapies for giving short shrift to affective processes ('hot' cognitions) while they focus primarily on the logic or rationality of clients' cognitions ('cold' cognitions). In some of these cognitive therapies, such as RET, there is the assumption that affect is largely 'postcognitive', namely that emotional reactions occur after perceptual and cognitive processing of information. The evidence suggests otherwise, however (Mahoney, 1980; Zajonc, 1980). Affective responses may be more fundamental, more rapid, and independent of cold cognitive judgments. According to Zajonc: 'affect and cognition are under the control of separate and partially independent systems that can influence each other in a variety of ways, and that both constitute independent sources of effects in information processing' (Zajonc, 1980, p. 151).

This concept of partially independent systems of psychological functioning has received considerable attention within the behaviour therapies as the three systems analysis of anxiety disorders (Lang, 1969; Rachman and Hodgson, 1980). Analysis of the triple response components of overt behaviour, physiological arousal, and self-report of anxiety is vital to effective assessment and treatment and it helps to order our observations about the nature and modification of anxiety disorders. However, this description of different response components is just that—it is not a theory that delineates the interactional dynamics among the three systems. Of the theories discussed above, self-efficacy is an attempt to conceptualize these interactive processes, although it has been criticized for a relative neglect of emotional arousal (Barlow and Mavissakalian, 1981).

An alternative view of the interactions among the triple response systems of behaviour, physiological arousal, and self-report that is also cognitive in nature is Lang's (1979) bioinformational theory of emotional imagery. In this propositional analysis, an image is seen as a conceptual network, the cognitive structure of which controls specific physiological responding and serves as a phototype for overt behavioural expression. The difference between this theory and previous conditioning theory analyses of imagery and conditioned autonomic responses, e.g. Wolpe's (1958) reciprocal inhibition theory, is obvious. Lang stresses that an image is not an internal stimulus to which the person responds (the former S–R conception of imagery in the behaviour therapies). Rather, the person generates a conceptual structure that contains both stimulus and response propositions. Behaviour change 'depends not on simple exposure to fear stimuli, but on the generation of the relevant affective cognitive structure, the prototype for overt behaviour, which is subsequently modified into a more functional form' (Lang, 1979, p. 501).

One of the advantages of this theory is that it provides an explanation for the variable effects of exposure therapies in the treatment of phobic and obsessive–compulsive clients. Only those who generate the relevant affective stimulus and response propositions will respond successfully (Lang et al., 1970). Those who are unable (or unwilling?) to accomplish this primary processing of affective information will show poorer outcomes. Since Lang (1979) has been able to train subjects to improve their generation of affective response propositions, a direct test of this assumption of the theory seems feasible.

Two other aspects of the theory warrant comment here. Lang has stated: 'Once you have (emotional processing) it is not clear whether the next step is to modify the structure of related behavioural acts, the visceral responses, or the semantic information in the network' (Lang, 1979 p. 515). The evidence, as I pointed out above, clearly indicates that phobic disorders are most effectively treated using performance-based techniques. How Lang's bioinformational theory would predict this remains to be shown. Finally, if one of the implications of this theory is that generating the greatest amount of arousal (anxiety) during therapy should produce the most behavioural change, as Barlow and Mavissakalian (1981) suggest, the theory is inconsistent with treatment outcome data showing no such relationship (Marks, 1978). In both of these instances self-efficacy theory makes predictions that receive greater support from the available literature.

In a related development, Rachman (1980) has put forward the concept of emotional processing in an attempt to integrate the diverse phenomena associated with abnormal fear, including its undue persistence, its apparently unprovoked recurrence, and its incubation, as well as obsessions, nightmares, and abnormal grief reactions. Rachman defines emotional processing as 'a process whereby emotional disturbances are absorbed, and decline to the extent that other experiences and behaviour can proceed without disruption' (Rachman, 1980, p. 51). Drawing from experimental and clinical findings, Rachman suggests specific stimulus, state, and personality factors that might either help or hinder emotional processing. If this working concept of emotional processing lacks the precision of Lang's theory of bioinformational processing, it also spans a far wider range of clinical phenomena. The potential advantages of this line of thinking include the welcome attempt to construct a unified account of different fear-related disorders and its greater compatibility with contemporary psychological theory and research than the rudimentary S–R accounts of specific fear responses and individual treatment techniques that have previously guided behavioural interventions.

CONCLUSION

During the 1950s and 1960s, the behaviour therapies developed within the framework of classical and operant conditioning principles that had originally served importantly to distinguish behaviour therapy from other clinical approaches. Over the course of the 1970s, this conceptual commitment to conditioning theory peaked out—some would say even waned. In part this change reflected the shift to more technological considerations governing the increasingly broad application of behavioural techniques that had been developed and refined during the previous period of growth. Moreover, as psychology 'went cognitive' during the 1970s, cognitive concepts inevitably were drawn upon to guide and explain treatment strategies.

The coming decade is likely to see a focus on integrative theoretical analyses of psychological functioning, geared in large part to conceptualizing the interactions among behavioural, physiological, and cognitive (semantic) systems. In contrast to earlier peripheralistic emphases, central mediating mechanisms such as cognitive appraisal and emotional processing will feature prominently in these theoretical analyses. A significant concern is the degree to which theoretical development will receive attention. At least in the USA the technological tide of the 1970s shows no sign of abating. Indeed, the signs point to an increasing emphasis on technological development within the field. Striking a constructive balance between the science and the practice of behaviour therapy will be necessary if the mutual benefits of progress within each domain are to be realized.

NOTES

1. Gone, however, is the once unbridled optimism about modifying any behaviour, the sense of which—with apologies to Archimedes—seemed to be: *'Give us an M and M big enough and a place to stand, and we can change any behaviour!'*.
2. Other applied behaviour analysts, a prominent example of whom is Azrin (1977), view the application of the existing behavioural technology to socially important problems as the preferred course of action. Similarly, Hayes *et al.* cite Risley's view that this decrease in conceptual analyses reflects 'the proper use of conductive methodology in behaviour analyses' (Hayes *et al.*, 1980 p. 283).
3. Bandura's is not the only social learning theory. Rotter (1954), for example, used the term 'social learning' as have other psychologists. Rosenthal (1981) points out that many developmental psychologists use the term in a broadly descriptive manner not identified with any particular lineage. Bandura's approach is distinctive, the one that has exercised the greatest influence within the behaviour therapies.
4. In fact, current cognitive behaviour therapies have little formal connection with modern cognitive psychology (Mahoney, 1980; Rosenthal, 1981).

REFERENCES

Abramson, L. Y., Seligman, M. E. P., and Teasdale, J. D. (1978) Learned helplessness in humans: Critique and reformulation. *Journal of Abnormal Psychology*, **87**, 49–74.
Agras, W. S., and Berkowitz, R. (1980) Clinical research in behavior therapy: Halfway there? *Behavior Therapy*, **11**, 472–487.
American Psychologist (1981) Toward the delineation of therapeutic change principles *American Psychologist*, (in press).
Azrin, N. H. (1977) A strategy for applied research: Learning based but outcome oriented. *American Psycholgist*, **32**, 140–149.
Bandura, A. (1969) *Principles of behavior modification*. Holt, New York.
Bandura, A. (1976) Self-reinforcement: Theoretical and methodological considerations. *Behaviorism*, **4**, 135–155.
Bandura, A. (1977a) Self-efficacy: Toward a unifying theory of behavioral change. *Psychological Review*, **84**, 191–215.
Bandura, A. (1977b) *Social learning theory*. Prentice-Hall, Englewood-Cliffs, New Jersey.
Bandura, A. (1978) Reflections on self-efficacy. *Advances in Behaviour Research and Therapy*, **1**, 237–269.

Bandura, A. (1980) The self and mechanisms of agency, in Suls, J., (ed.) *Social psychological perspectives on the self.* Erlbaum, Hillsdale, New Jersey.

Bandura, A., Adams, N., Hardy, A., and Howells, G. (1980). Tests of the generality of self-efficacy theory. *Cognitive Therapy and Research,* **4,** 39–66.

Barlow, D. H., and Mavissakalian, M. R. (1981). Directions in the assessment and treatment of phobia: The next decade, in Mavissakalian, M. R., and Barlow, D. H., (eds.), *Phobia: Psychological and pharmacological treatment,* Guilford Press, New York, (in press).

Barrios, B. (1979) The role of self-efficacy in the reduction of heterosocial anxiety: A microanalysis. *Paper presented at Association for Advancement of Behavior Therapy,* San Francisco.

Beck, A. T. (1976) *Cognitive therapy and the emotional disorders,* International Universities Press, New York.

Bersh, P. J. (1980) Eysenck's theory of incubation. *Behaviour Research and Therapy,* **18,** 11–18.

Biran, M., and Wilson, G. T. (1980) Participant modeling versus cognitive restructuring in the treatment of phobic disorders. *Paper presented at World Congress on Bahavior Therapy,* Jerusalem, July, 1980.

Boulougouris, C. J. and Rabavilas, A.: (eds.). (1977) *The Treatment of Phobic and Obsessive–Compulsive Disorders.* Pergamon Press, Oxford.

Bower, G. (1978) Contacts of cognitive psychology with social learning theory. *Cognitive Therapy and Research,* **2,** 2.

Breger, L., and McGaugh, J. L. (1966) A critique and reformulation of 'learning theory' approaches to psychotherapy and neurosis. *Psychological Bulletin,* **65,** 170–173.

Brewer, W. F. (1974) There is no convincing evidence for operant or classical conditioning in adult humans, in Weiner, W and Palermo, D. (eds.), *Cognition and the symbolic processes,* Erlbaum, Hillsdale, New Jersey, pp. 1–42.

Butcher, J. N., and Koss, M. P. (1978) Research on brief and crisis-oriented psychotherapies, in Garfield, S. L., and Bergin, A. E. (eds.), *Handbook of psychotherapy and behavior change.* Wiley, New York, pp. 725–767.

Catania, A. C. (1975) The myth of self-reinforcement. *Behaviorism,* **3,** 192–199.

Collins, R. L. (1980) *The comparative efficacy of cognitive and behavioral approaches to obesity.* Doctoral dissertation, Rutgers University.

Condiotti, M., and Lichtenstein, E. (1980) *Self-efficacy and relapse in smoking cessation programs.* Unpublished manuscript, University of Oregon.

Cooney, N. L. (1980) *Coping with relapse: A social learning approach to preventing smoking recidivism.* Masters thesis, Rutgers University.

Craighead, E., Kimball, W., and Rehak, P. (1979) Mood changes, physiological responses and self-statements during social rejection imagery. *Journal of Consulting and Clinical Psychology,* **47,** 385–396.

Deitz, S. M. (1978) Current status of applied behavior analysis: Science versus technology. *American Psychologist,* **33,** 805–814.

Delprato, D. J. (1980) Hereditary determinants of fears and phobias: a critical review. *Behavior Therapy,* **11,** 79–103.

DeSilva, P., Rachman, S., and Seligman, M. E. P. Prepared phobias and obsessions: therapeutic outcome. *Behaviour Research and Therapy,* **15,** 65–77.

DiClemente, C. C. (1981) Self-efficacy and smoking cessation maintenance. *Cognitive Therapy and Research,* (in press).

Ellis, A. (1977) Rejoinder: Elegant and inelegant RET. *The Counselling Psychologist* **7,** 73–82.

Erwin, E. (1978) *Behavior Therapy.* Cambridge University Press, New York.

Eysenck, H. E. (1960) *Behaviour therapy and the neuroses.* Pergamon Press, Oxford.

Eysenck, H. J. (1970) Behavior therapy and its critics. *Journal of Behavior Therapy and Experimental Psychiatry*, **1**, 5–15.

Eysenck, H. J. (1979) Behavior therapy and the philosophers. *Behaviour Research and Therapy*, **17**, 511–514.

Eysenck, H. J. (1981) The neo-behavioristic (S–R) theory of behavior therapy, in Wilson, G. T. and Franks, C. M. (eds.), *Handbook of behavior therapy*. Guilford Press, New York, (in press).

Foreyt, J., and Rathjen, D. (1978) *Cognitive behavior therapy: Research and application*. Plenum Press, New York.

Franks, C. M., and Wilson, G. T. (1977) *Annual review of behavior therapy: Theory and practice*, Brunner/Mazel, New York. Vol. 5.

Franks, C. M., and Wilson, G. T. (1978) *Annual review of behavior therapy: Theory and practice*, Brunner/Mazel, New York. Vol. 6.

Franks, C. M., and Wilson, G. T. (1979) *Annual review of behavior therapy: Theory and practice*, Brunner/Mazel, New York. Vol. 7.

Goldfried, M. R., and Davison, G. C. (1976) *Clinical behavior therapy*, Holt, Rinehart & Winston, New York.

Goldiamond, I. (1976) Fables, armadyllics, and self-reinforcement. *Journal of Applied Behavior Analysis*, **9**, 521–525.

Hayes, S. C., Rincover, A., and Solnick, J. (1980) The technical drift of applied behavior analysis. *Journal of Applied Behavior Analysis*, **13**, 275–286.

Herrnstein, R. J. (1969) Method and theory in the study of avoidance. *Psychological Review*, **76**, 46–69.

Hersen, M., and Barlow, D. H. (1976) *Single-case experimental designs: Strategies for studying behavior change*. Pergamon Press, New York.

Hugdahl, K. (1978) Electrodermal conditioning to potentially phobic stimuli: Effects of instructed extinction. *Behaviour Research and Therapy*, **16**, 315–321.

Hygge, S., and Ohman, A. (1978) Modelling processes in the acquisition of fears: Vicarious electrodermal conditioning to fear-relevant stimuli. *Journal of Personality and Social Psychology*, **36**, 271–279.

Jacobson, N. S. (1978) A review of the research on the effectiveness of marital therapy, in Paolino, T. J., and McCrady, B. S. (eds.), *Marriage and marital therapy*. Brunner/Mazel, New York, pp. 395–444.

Jacobson, N., and Weiss, R. (1978) Behavioral marriage therapy: III. The contents of Gurman *et al.* may be hazardous to our health. *Family Process*, **17**, 149–163.

Kazdin, A. E. (1978) The application of operant techniques in treatment, rehabilitation, and education, in Garfield, S. L., and Bergin, (eds.), *Handbook of psychotherapy and behavior change*, (2nd edn.) Wiley, New York.

Kazdin, A. E., and Wilson, G. T. (1978) *Evaluation of behavior therapy: Issues, evidence and research strategies*. Ballinger, Cambridge, Mass.

Knudson, R. M., Gurman, A. S., and Kniskern, D. P. (1979) Behavioral marriage therapy: A treatment in transition, in Franks, C. M., and Wilson, G. T., (eds.), *Annual review of behavior therapy: Theory and practice*, Brunner/Mazel, New York, Vol. 7, pp. 543–574.

Lang, P. E. (1969) The mechanics of desensitization and the laboratory study of fear, in Franks, C. M. (ed.), *Behavior therapy: Appraisal and status*. McGraw-Hill, New York, pp. 160–191.

Lang, P. J. (1979) A bioinformational theory of emotional imagery. *Psychophysiology*, **16**, 495–512.

Lang, P. J., Melamed, B. G., (1970) Hart, J. A psychophysiological analysis of fear modification using an automated desensitization procedure. *Journal of Abnormal Psychology*, **76**, 220–234.

Leitenberg, H. (1976) *Handbook of behavior modification and behavior therapy*, Prentice-Hall, Englewood Cliffs, New Jersey.

London, P. (1972) The end of ideology in behavior modification, *American Psychologist*, **27**, 913–926.

Mahoney, M. J. (1974) *Cognition and behavior modification*, Ballinger, Cambridge, Mass.

Mahoney, M. J. (1980) Psychotherapy and the structure of personal revolutions, in Mahoney, M. J. (ed.), *Cognition and clinical science*, Plenum, New York.

Mahoney, M. J., and Arnkoff, D. (1978) Cognitive and self-control therapies, in Garfield, S. L., and Bergin, A. E., (eds.), *Handbook of psychotherapy and behavior change*, (2nd edn.) Wiley, New York, pp. 689–722.

Marks, I. (1978) Behavioral psychotherapy of adult neurosis, in Garfield, S. L., and Bergin, A. E., (eds.), *Handbook of psychotherapy and behavior change*, (2nd edn.) Wiley, New York, pp. 493–548.

Marlatt, G. A., and Gordon, J. R. (1979) Determinants of relapse: Implications for the maintenance of behavior change, in Davidson, P., and Davidson, S., (eds.), *Behavioral medicine: Changing health lifestyles*. Brunner/Mazel, New York, pp. 410–452.

McLean, P. D., and Hakstian, A. R. (1979) Clinical depression: comparative efficacy of outpatient treatments. *Journal of Consulting and Clinical Psychology*, **47**, 818–836.

Meichenbaum, D. (1977) *Cognitive behavior modification*. Plenum, New York.

Meichenbaum, D. and Cameron, R. (1981) Cognitive behavior modification: Current issues, in Wilson, G. T., and Franks, C. M. (eds.), *Handbook of behavior therapy*. Guilford Press, New York, (in press).

Miller, W. R. (ed.) (1981) *The addictive behaviors: Treatment of alcoholism, drug abuse, smoking and obesity*. Pergamon Press, New York, (in press).

Mowrer, O. H. (1960) *Learning theory and behavior*. Wiley, New York.

O'Leary, K. D., and Turkewitz, H. (1978) Marital therapy from a behavioral perspective, in Paolino, T. J., and McCrady, B. S. (eds.), *Marriage and marital therapy*. Brunner/Mazel, New York, pp. 240–297.

Paul, G. L., and Lentz, R. J. (1977) *Psychosocial treatment of chronic mental patients: Milieu versus social-learning programs*. Harvard University Press, Cambridge, Mass.

Perlmuter, L. C., and Monty, R. A. (eds.) (1980) *Choice and perceived control*. Erlbaum, Hillsdale, New Jersey.

Rabavilas, A. D., Boulougouris, J. C., and Stefanis, C. (1976) Duration of flooding sessions in the treatment of obsessive–compulsive patients. *Behaviour Research and Therapy*, **14**, 349–355.

Rachlin, H. (1976) *Behavior and learning*. Freeman, San Francisco, Ca.

Rachlin, H. (1977) A review of M. J. Mahoney's *Cognition and Behavior Modification*. *Journal of Applied Behavior Analysis*, **10**, 369–374.

Rachman, S. (1976) The passing of the two-stage theory of fear and avoidance: Fresh possibilities. *Behaviour Research and Therapy*, **14**, 125–131.

Rachman, S. (1977) The conditioning theory of fear-acquisition: an initial examination. *Behaviour Research and Therapy*, **15**, 375–388.

Rachman, S. (ed.) (1978) Perceived self-efficacy: Analyses of Bandura's theory of behavioral change. *Advances in Behaviour Research and Therapy*, **1**, 139–269.

Rachman, S. (1980) Emotional processing. *Behaviour Research and Therapy*, **18**, 51–60.

Rachman, S., and Hodgson, R. (1980) *Obsessions and compulsions*. Prentice-Hall, Englewood Cliffs, New Jersey.

Rachman, S., and Wilson, G. T. (1980) *Effects of psychotherapy*, Pergamon Press, Oxford.

Rescorla, R., and Wagner, A. (1972) A theory of Pavlovian conditioning, in Black, A., and Prokasy, W. (eds.), *Classical conditioning*, Appleton-Century-Crofts, New York, Vol. 2, pp. 64–99.

Rescorla, R., and Solomon, R. (1967) Two-process learning theory: Relationships between Pavlovian conditioning and instrumental learning. *Psychological Review*, **74**, 151–182.

Rodin, J. (1978) Cognitive-behavioral strategies for the control of obesity, in Meichenbaum, D. (ed.), *Cognitive behavior therapy*. BMA Audio Cassette Publications, New York.

Rosenthal, B. S., and Marx, R. D. (1979) A comparison of standard behavioural and relapse prevention weight reduction programs. *Paper presented at Association of Advancement of Behavior Therapy*, San Francisco.

Rosenthal, T. L. (1981) On the significance of differences between social learning theory and cognitive-behavioral conceptions: Type I and Type II errors, in Wilson, G. T. and Franks, C. M. (eds.), *Handbook of behavior therapy*. Guilford Press, New York (in press).

Rosenthal, T. L., and Bandura, A. (1978) Psychological modeling: Theory and practice, in Garfield, S. L., and Bergin, A. E. (eds.), *Handbook of psychotherapy and behavior change* (2nd edn.) Wiley, New York, pp. 621–658.

Rosenthal, T. L., and Zimmerman, B. J. (1978) *Social learning and cognition*. Academic Press, New York.

Rotter, J. B. (1954) *Social learning and clinical psychology*, Prentice-Hall, Englewood Cliffs, New Jersey.

Rush, A. J., Beck, A. T., Kovacs, M., and Hollon, S. (1977) Comparative efficacy of cognitive therapy and pharmacotherapy in the treatment of depressed outpatients. *Cognitive Therapy and Research*, **1**, 17–37.

Seligman, M. E. P. (1971) Phobias and preparedness. *Behavior Therapy*, **2**, 307–320.

Seligman, M. E. P. (1975) *Helplessness*, Freeman, San Francisco, Ca.

Thibaut, J. W., and Kelley, H. H. (1959) *The social psychology of groups*, Wiley, New York.

Ullmann, L. P., and Krasner, L. (1975) *A psychological approach to abnormal behavior*, (2nd edn.) Prentice-Hall, Englewood Cliffs, New Jersey.

Weiss, R. (1979) Resistance in behavioral marriage therapy. *The American Journal of Family Therapy*, **3**, 3–6.

Williams, S., and Rappoport, A. (1980) *Behavioral practice with and without cognitive modification in agoraphobics*. Unpublished manuscript, Stanford University.

Wilson, G. T. (1973) Counterconditioning versus forced exposure in extinction of avoidance responding and conditioned fear in rats. *Journal of Comparative and Physiological Psychology*, **82**, 105–116.

Wilson, G. T. (1978a) Booze, beliefs and behavior: Cognitive factors in alcohol use and abuse, in Nathan, P. E., Marlatt, G. A., and Loberg, T., (eds.), *Alcoholism: New directions in behavioral research and treatment*. Plenum, New York, pp. 315–339.

Wilson, G. T. (1978b) The importance of being theoretical: Comments on Bandura's 'Self-efficacy: Toward a unifying theory of behavioral change'. *Advances in Behaviour Research and Therapy*, **1**, 217–230.

Wilson, G. T., and Brownell, K. (1980) *Behavior therapy for obesity: An evaluation of treatment outcome*. Unpublished manuscript, Rutgers University.

Wilson, G. T., and O'Leary, K. D. (1980) *Principles of behavior therapy*, Prentice-Hall, Englewood Cliffs, New Jersey.

Wolpe, J. (1958) *Psychotherapy by reciprocal inhibition*. Stanford University Press, Stanford.

Wolpe, J. (1976) Behaviour therapy and its malcontents—II. Multimodal exlecticism, cognitive exclusivism and 'exposure' empiricism. *Journal of Behavior Therapy and Experimental Psychiatry*, **7**, 109–116.

Wooley, S. C., Wooley, O. W., and Dyrenforth, S. T. (1979) Theoretical, practical, and social issues in behavioral treatments of obesity. *Journal of Applied Behavior Analysis*, **12**, 3–25.

Zajonc, R. (1980) Feeling and thinking. *American Psychologist*, **35**, 151–175.

Learning Theory Approaches to Psychiatry
Edited by John Boulougouris
© 1982 John Wiley & Sons Ltd

4. WHAT KIND OF THEORY WILL IMPROVE PSYCHOLOGICAL TREATMENT?

John Teasdale

When invited to contribute to this book I was asked to discuss (1) the relevance of learning theory models to the behavioural therapies applied to psychiatric patients; (2) the inadequecies of these models; and (3) what needs to be done in order to understand better the psychiatric patient and to find more effective procedures. Emboldened by such wide terms of reference I thought it would be interesting to try to answer the third of these questions as it is at once both the most difficult and most important. It seemed consistent with the spirit of the other questions to look for guidance on this issue to the relationship of learning theory models to the development of effective behavioural treatments. Historically, this appears to have been a very productive relationship. What would we learn from the application of the basic paradigms of operant and classical conditioning to the development of treatment that might better inform our development of new treatment procedures? History will always defy any single interpretation and so the search for the lessons of history in this area is necessarily an exercise in speculation rather than science. It may, none the less, be worthwhile.

THE LESSONS OF HISTORY

In attempting to develop a psychological treatment for a clinical condition we need to answer a series of questions something like those shown in Table 1. This Table indicates how the operant and classical conditioning paradigms have provided useful answers to these questions for two clinical problems, phobias and the self-mutilatory behaviour of headbanging. The initial questions to be asked: 'How should I conceptualize this problem? What in principle does my conceptualization suggest needs doing?' are those which would be considered in making a behavioural analysis of the problem. Answering them requires resort to a theory of some sort. However, this theory may not be of a very sophisticated or detailed nature. In fact, the type of theory which seems to have guided the development of behavioural treatments often seems to have been of the simple form: 'Let us look at clinical

Table 1. Questions asked in developing a psychological treatment

	Phobias: Answers from the classical conditioning paradigm.	Headbanging: Answers from the operant conditioning paradigm
A.	How should I conceptualize this problem? Which of its many features should I focus on?	Regard the phobia as a conditioned fear. Focus on the autonomic and other responses elicited by presentation of the phobic stimuli, and the passive avoidance behaviour resulting from this conditioned fear	Regard the headbanging as a positively reinforced operant. Focus on the immediate reinforcing consequences contingent on the response
B.	What in principle does my conceptualization of the problem suggest needs doing?	Extinguish fear conditioned to the CS	Extinguish the positively reinforced operant
C.	How in practice is this to be achieved?	Repeatedly present the phobic stimulus in the absence of any aversive UCSs	Identify and withhold the reinforcing consequences of headbanging (instruct nurses to withhold attention).
D.	How can I measure whether I have affected the changes I was aiming for?	Measure autonomic and other responses to presentation of phobic stimuli; and changes in approach behaviour to phobic stimuli	Count the frequency of headbanging behaviours and attentional reinforcers within a reversal design

problem X as if aspects of it were similar to the behaviour we have studied in our laboratory paradigm Y'. This type of theory allows us to derive possible methods of intervention for our clinical problem from the empirical generalizations established by studying a variety of experimental manipulations within paradigm Y.

It should be stressed that this type of approach does not depend on any detailed theoretical understanding of the mechanisms underlying the phenomena studied in the laboratory paradigm. Hypotheses concerning the process of classical conditioning have changed radically since the time of Pavlov, but this has not affected some of the basic empirical generalizations which can be made concerning the effects of repeatedly pairing and unpairing stimuli in different ways. It is these in which we are primarily interested in a low level theory of the form: 'Let us look at X as if it were similar to aspects of Y'. Indeed, as has often been pointed out, the basic 'theories' underlying the operant and classical conditioning paradigms were by no means novel; learning by association and the notion that behaviour is affected by its consequences have been aspects of common knowledge for some considerable time. The advance in scientific knowledge that the operant and classical conditioning paradigms have produced has not depended on the resurrection of such basic 'theories'. Rather, it has resulted from the fact that they have developed as scientific paradigms (Kuhn, 1962), which involve much more than theoretical statements. A scientific paradigm provides an organizational focus around which, by concentrating on certain key experimental situations, a body of related and integrated knowledge and a methodology of investigation and measurement can be developed. It involves far more than theory. The history of science suggest that knowledge accumulates most rapidly when the investigations of different scientists can be integrated by their relationship to a shared paradigm (Kuhn, 1962). While theory is an important aspect of a paradigm it is only one of a number of components.

I would suggest that something similar is probably true of the place of theory in the development of behavioural treatments from application of the operant and classical conditioning paradigms. That is, the creation of successful treatment methods depended as much on the fact that operant and classical conditioning were fairly well-developed scientific paradigms as on theories of learning as such. As we suggested above, the single most important theoretical exercise in the development of the behavioural treatments was the imaginative leap of regarding aspects of clinical problems as similar to behaviours studied within these established paradigms. Once this step had been taken it was possible to draw on the accumulated wealth of empirical generalizations and experimental and measurement methodology which had been established within the paradigms of operant and classical conditioning. The importance of this step can be illustrated by considering how we might answer questions C and D in Table 1. These ask how we are actually going to achieve the desired change in the clinical condition and how we are going to measure whether we have achieved the end for which we were aiming. Theory is of limited assistance here. Thus, for example, regarding a phobia as if it were a classically conditioned fear response does not by itself tell us how we are to reduce the intensity of the conditioned fear. The important step here is that, having once regarded the phobia as a classically conditioned response, we can look for guidance to the wealth of empirical generalizations established within the classical conditioning paradigm. This tells us that one way to reduce the intensity of a conditioned response is to present repeatedly the conditioned stimulus in the absence of the unconditioned stimulus. This can be translated quite directly into a method of treatment that can be tried out on clinical phobias. It is also possible to draw on the measurement methodology established within the experimental paradigm for suggestions as to how to measure the variables the paradigm suggest are important.

One lesson of history appears to be that the development of effective behavioural treatments depended not so much on their derivation from 'learning theories' as from established scientific paradigms, with all that that involves. It could also be argued that following the introduction of behavioural treatments their further development has progressed most rapidly where investigations have been organized in structures approaching paradigms within the applied field itself. Applied behavioural analysis and analogue phobia research spring to mind as examples. While the exact relevance of the latter to the treatment of clinical phobias has been often debated, I am in no doubt that this line of research, which includes many conceptually and empirically related investigations, has contributed very usefully to the evolution of more effective treatment for phobias.

The paradigmatic status of operant and classical conditioning has been an important factor contributing to the successful development of behavioural treatments. However, clearly this by itself is not sufficient; the paradigms also have to be relevant to the nature and treatment of the clinical problems in which we are interested. How can we assess relevance?

The most obvious test of relevance is whether the paradigm can generate effective treatments. However, it is clearly desirable to have some other basis on which to select paradigms before examining in detail their therapeutic potential. One possible basis is whether the paradigm appears able to provide a plausible account of the origins and maintenance of the clinical condition in which we are interested. Interestingly, it appears that a paradigm need not necessarily provide a valid account of the origins of a clinical condition for it to be able to generate effective treatments. One of the weakest aspects of the conditioned fear model of phobias is the difficulty in identifying an initial pairing of the phobic stimulus with a traumatic event in the origin of many phobias. Similarly, it is difficult to maintain that the principles of operant conditioning, which are of considerable value in the management of psychotic and mentally handicapped individuals, can be themselves give an adequate account of the initial causes of the pathology of these individuals.

The ability to provide a convincing account of the origins of a disorder does not appear to be a necessary requirement of relevance for a paradigm. By contrast, the ability to provide a plausible account of the current state and maintenance of the disorder does. This appears true of the successful applications of the operant and classical conditioning paradigms we have been considering. The absence of this feature also seems to characterize some of the unsuccessful applications of these paradigms. One of the more obvious of these has been the relative failure of aversion therapy to produce clinically useful results in the treatment of alcoholism. In this case the treatment method was clearly derived from the classical conditioning paradigm and attempted to condition unpleasant feelings to alcohol-related stimuli. However, the method of treatment was not linked to a plausible account of the maintenance of alcoholism derived from this paradigm. It is, of course, possible to suggest that excessive drinking is maintained by unusually strong positive emotional responses conditioned to alcohol-related stimuli so that treatment should be directed at modifying these responses. However, this suggestion hardly seems to do justice to the clinical facts we have.

How are we to assess the adequacy with which a paradigm can provide an account of the maintenance of a clinical condition? One method is, as in the preceding section, simply to make a judgement of its face validity or plausibility. A preferable approach would be to conduct more detailed experimental investigations of the account of the condition's psychopathology which has been derived from the paradigm. One line of enquiry would be to explore the account's predictions concerning the effect of various interventions on the symptomatology of the clinical condition. Ethical contraints will probably proscribe investigations of interventions predicted to increase clinical symptomatology. Study is more likely to be directed at experimental manipulations predicted to reduce symptoms. These have the added advantage that they might well produce information of direct relevance to the development of treatments. They thus offer a double pay-off, both to increasing understanding of the condition and to treatment development. These investigations might well take the form of therapy analogue studies, either looking at the effects of short-term interventions in clinical conditions or of longer-term interventions in milder non-clinical conditions. Compared to full-scale trials of clinical treatments such studies benefit from the greater precision with which interventions can be specified and their effects measured. They are also more economical.

Accepting the severe constraints on the historical exercise we have undertaken, how can we summarize the lessons we can tentatively draw from the history of the development of behavioural treatments? First, it is an advantage if we can look for guidance in the development of treatments to established scientific paradigms. Second, such paradigms should be able to offer acceptable account of the maintenance, if not the origins, of the clinical condition which we are interested in treating. In other words, our treatment should be related to an acceptable account of the condition's psychopathology. Third, a valuable approach to assessing the validity of the paradigm-derived account is to study the effects of experimental interventions predicted by the account to reduce symptomatology.

What happens when we apply these lessons from history to the present, specifically to attempts to develop psychological treatments for a condition which is not comfortably handled within the classical and operant conditioning paradigms, depression?

THE LESSONS OF HISTORY APPLIED TO TREATMENTS FOR DEPRESSION

It would not be unfair to characterize the current status of psychological accounts and treatments for depression as 'much theory, few paradigms'. From our previous discussion this would suggest that there should be no shortage of answers to the first two questions in Table 1, namely, how to conceptualize the nature of the problem and what in principle to do about it. However, it would suggest we might be short of tried and tested ways of implementing the changes that our theoretical statements suggest are required, and of ways of measuring the effects of those changes. Further, it is likely that our theoretical statements will be short of empirical support.

Currently we have a range of interesting psychological theories of depression. Each has a little empirical work to support it but none of these areas of investigation approaches the status of a scientific paradigm. Similarly, there are a number of approaches to the psychological treatment of depression for which the preliminary evidence of effectiveness is encouraging. Some of these treatments are related to theories of the nature of depression. However, at the moment we have no evidence that these treatments actually operate through the specific mechanisms the theories to which they relate would suggest. As the treatments themselves are often quite complex packages it is probable that their further refinement and improvement will depend on identification of such specific mechanisms.

What guidance do the lessons of history offer to the further improvement of psychological treatments of depression? The first recommendation is that our treatments should be related to a relevant experimental paradigm. Of the various psychological accounts of depression currently popular the learned helplessness approach (Seligman, 1975; Abramson et al., 1978) is the most obviously paradigm-related. Examining the strengths and weaknesses of this approach may be instructive.

While learned helplessness is obviously not so well established as a scientific paradigm as operant or classical conditioning there already exists a considerable body of inter-related theory, experimental findings and investigative methodology in this area. Thus, learned helplessness approximates the first criterion required by the lessons of history. How does learned helplessness score on the criterion that the paradigm should be relevant to the clinical condition, in this case depression? In other words, how valid is the claim that learned helplessness offers a model of clinical depression (Seligman, 1975) particularly with respect to the maintenance of the condition? There is no generally accepted answer to this question, as anyone familiar with the special issue of the *Journal of Abnormal Psychology* devoted to this topic will be aware (*Journal of Abnormal Psychology*, February 1978). One of the major reservations concerns the extent to which parallels between clinical symptomatology and the experimentally investigated phenomena are convincing.for example, do the deficits in anagram or shuttlebox performance typically studied in laboratory studies of human helplessness have any relation to the widespread behavioural and motivational deficits in clinical depression? Similarly, can explanations in terms of reduced expectancy of success proposed to account for deficits on such novel laboratory tasks convincingly account for the deficits patients show on everyday overlearned tasks such as bedmaking, speech, or social interaction? Space precludes the discussion of such issues in any detail here. It is sufficient for our present purpose to say that, at the level of face validity, the relevance of the phenomena investigated in laboratory studies of learned helplessness if far from universally accepted. If face validity can offer no generally agreed answer to the question whether learned helplessness is relevant to clinical depression what of experimental investigations testing predictions of the model directly in the clinical condition? Earlier it was suggested that investigating experimental manipulations predicted to reduce symptomatology would be a particularly useful method of enquiry. Unfortunately no such investigations of the learned helplessness account appear to have been published as yet. Thus, although the learned helplessness approach to depression relates to a body of experimental literature, the relevance of this to the clinical condition is not clearly established. How does this affect the answers that could be given to the questions posed in Table 1 by the learned helplessness approach to depression at the present time? In response to the questions: 'How should I conceptualize this problem? Which of its many features should I focus on?' this approach suggests that maintenance of depression should be conceptualized as effects in a number of response systems resulting from expectations of uncontrollable loss (Abramson *et al.*, 1978) and attention should be focused on these expectations. As we have just indicated, the validity of this conceptualization has yet to be established. The answer to the second question: 'What in principle does my conceptualization of the problem suggest needs doing?' follows clearly from the answer to the first: change the expectations of uncontrollable loss. Abramson *et al.* (1978) have developed a more detailed answer to this question indicating how, in principle, this end might be achieved by changing the perceived probabilities of aversive or desired outcomes, reducing the aversiveness of highly aversive outcomes or the desirability of highly desired outcomes, changing expectations from uncontrollability to controllability, and changing unrealistic attributions for failure and success experiences. While our conceptualization gives us reasonably clear goals of what, in principle, needs to be done, work within the learned helplessness approach has relatively little to offer in the way of more specific means for achieving these goals. We know that learned helplessness in dogs, manifested as deficits in shuttlebox escape–avoidance, can be alleviated by dragging the dog backwards and forwards across the shuttlebox so that it is exposed to the contingency that shock terminates as it crosses the barrier (Seligman *et al.*, 1968). We also know that successfully solving cognitive problems can alleviate the deficits in shuttlebox and anagram performance shown by helpless students and the deficits in shuttlebox performance shown by mildly depressed students (Klein and Seligman, 1976; Teasdale, 1978). However, the direct relevance of this to the development of interventions in clinical depression is somewhat limited. So, the current contribution of the learned helplessness approach to answering question C in Table 1 is rather low.

Much the same is true when we consider the question of how to measure clinically the variables held to be important by the learned helplessness approach, and to measure the effects of interventions derived from this approach. The measurement of expectations of control of outcomes is not particularly well developed within the experimental methodology of learned helplessness. Further, the main dependent variables which have been studied within the laboratory studies of learned helplessness, performance on tasks such as shuttlebox escape–avoidance or anagram solution, are quite removed from the variables commonly used to measure clinical depression. For this reason the experimental studies have contributed relatively little to the methodology of measuring the effect of treatment interventions on outcome.

In summary, we may say that the learned helplessness approach offers both a way of conceptualizing clinical depression and a range of suggestions of how, in principle, depression might be treated. The validity of this conceptualization has yet to be firmly established, and so the treatment suggestions must be used with caution. Work within the learned helplessness approach has so far been of limited assistance in suggesting specific methods of intervention in clinical depression, and in providing a methodology of measurement with much relevance to the clinical situation. Much the same could be said of other currently popular psychological approaches to depression. In general these have a smaller body of related investigation to draw on than the learned helplessness approach.

'Many theories, few paradigms' seems a fair description of the current state of psychological approaches to understanding and treating depression. However, to expect paradigmatic status in this area is to have high expectations indeed; established scientific paradigms are quite rare in psychology as a whole, and the interest of empirically-oriented psychologists in depression is a very recent development. It may well be that, with time, paradigms with relevance to treatment will evolve in this area. As we are not yet at this point it may be useful to consider some of the alternative routes forward in the development of psychological treatments for depression, in the light of the lessons of history.

One currently popular approach is to take a psychological theory of depression, to work out its prescriptions for treatment, to design a treatment package, often complex, to realize these, and then to evaluate the over-all clinical effectiveness of this package. This approach has had the virtue of producing packages that, in terms of the early evidence available, seem to be effective in producing greater reduction in depression than no treatment. The disadvantage of this approach is that as the treatments are often complex and outcome is often only assessed with relatively crude measures, this approach does little to increase our understanding of the nature of depression or of the means by which the treatments were effective. History suggests that such understanding is likely to be of great benefit in increasing treatment effectiveness and efficiency. There is always the possibility, of course, of disassembling complex treatment packages in order to identify their active ingredients. The difficulty here is that if, as some have suggested, the effective ingredients in the treatment of depression are things like the elicitation of hope for change, this may depend on a complex interaction of the constituent parts of the whole. In this case, disassembly studies may yield less clear cut results than, for example, the studies which examined the effects of removing the relaxation component from the systematic desensitization treatment of phobias.

A second approach is to throw our resources into 'basic' psychological research into the nature of depression, possibly establishing scientific paradigms in the course of this. If this work gave us a sounder understanding of depression than we have at the moment, we would be able to answer the first two questions in Table 1 with much more confidence than we can at present. This would give us a much firmer foundation from which to develop treatments. However, 'basic' research would not necessarily provide us with answers to the third and fourth questions in Table 1, how in practice to achieve change, and how to measure the process and effects of change.

A third approach is to conduct experimental investigations of clearly defined interventions which are predicted by theoretical models to reduce the symptomatology of clinical depression. Such investigations would simultaneously constitute both 'basic' research, in testing theoretical predictions, and 'analogue therapy' research in providing suggestions for the components of more complex treatment packages. They offer the possibility of providing more firmly based theories from which to answer the first two questions in Table 1. They would also provide answers to the third question in that Table. This kind of study would depend on the development of more precise measures of depression and of aspects of the intervention process, and so would contribute answers to the fourth question in Table 1. In the development of behavioural treatments, analogue phobia research, and some of the work within applied behavioural analysis approximate the type of work that would be included in this type of approach. In depression, the 'spontaneous' variability of the condition poses more problems than with phobias, suggesting that investigations might have to be intensive rather than extensive over time.

The arguments for the third approach seems strong, and are, of course, by no means novel. One of the major difficulties in implementing this approach at present is the lack of a clear description or definition of the dependent variable, the state of depression, and of means of measuring it more precisely. As these are likely to be obstacles to the development of better understanding and treatment of depression anyway, adoption of this strategy would apply welcome pressure to resolve rather than by-pass these difficulties.

CONCLUSION

How should we answer the question posed in the title? First, we want a theory that provides an integrated account of the maintenance of the clinical condition we wish to treat and of the means of treating it. Second, we want a theory with considerable empirical support so that our treatments have a firm foundation. Third, there are considerable advantages if our theory can be paradigm-related. This increases the chances of the theory having a body of supporting experimental data. Further, it makes it more likely that we can look to relevant experimentation for guidance on how to effect change and how to measure it. Experimental investigation of the effects on clinical conditions of simple interventions, predicted by theory to reduce symptomatology, contribute to improving treatment in two ways. They improve theory development and, more directly, contribute to the methodology of achieving change and measuring its effects.

ACKNOWLEDGEMENT

The author is supported by a grant from the Medical Research Council of the United Kingdom.

REFERENCES

Abramson, L. Y., Seligman, M. E. P., and Teasdale, J. D. (1978) Learned helplessness in humans: critique and reformulation. *Journal of Abnormal Psychology*, **87**, 49–74.

Klein, D. C., and Seligman, M. E. P. (1976) Reversal of performance deficits in learned helplessness and depression. *Journal of Abnormal Psychology*, **85**, 11–26.

Kuhn, T. S. (1962) *The structure of scientific revolutions*, University of Chicago Press, Chicago.

Seligman, M. E. P. (1975) *Helplessness: On depression, development and death*. Freeman, San Francisco.

Seligman, M. E. P., Maier, S. F., and Geer, J. (1968) The alleviation of learned helplessness in the dog. *Journal of Abnormal and Social Psychology*, **73**, 256–262.

Teasdale, J. D. (1978) Effects of real and recalled success on learned helplessness and depression. *Journal of Abnormal Psychology*, **87**, 155–164.

Learning Theory Approaches to Psychiatry
Edited by John Boulougouris
© 1982 John Wiley & Sons Ltd

5. BIOFEEDBACK, PLACEBOS, AND LEARNING THEORY

Edward S. Katkin

Psychotherapy (as well as pharmacomedical therapy) is notorious for having non-specific, or placebo, effects; biofeedback (a specific form of psychotherapy), indeed, has been viewed by some researchers in the field as 'the ultimate placebo' (Stroebel and Glueck, 1973). Whether biofeedback treatment has specific therapeutic qualities that can be shown to be independent of demand characteristics, therapist bias, subject expectancy, base rates of spontaneous remission, and other non-specific factors must be demonstrated through properly controlled studies.

Strictly speaking, the concept of 'placebo' refers to the use of a pharmacologically inactive agent which is administered to a patient for a variety of reasons including the failure to identify a diagnosable disorder. Often, but not always, the placebo administration results in symptom reduction. It is not the case that a treatment is classified as a placebo because its mechanism is not understood; rather, it is classified as a placebo precisely when its mechanism is well-understood and there is no pharmacologically valid reason for it to succeed.

In the area of psychotherapy, the term placebo has been borrowed from medicine and employed frequently. In the psychotherapeutic sense, therefore, a placebo should refer to a type of treatment that is known to have no valid specific treatment effect, but which superficially appears to the patient to be an active form of psychotherapy. In other words, placebo psychotherapy should look like therapy, should sound like therapy, and should cause the patient to expect that he is receiving therapy. Nevertheless, the treatment should be understood to have no valid theoretical mechanism by which it could actually be therapy.

When one takes the definition of placebo seriously, it becomes apparent than an attempt to evaluate the effectiveness of traditional psychotherapy against placebo effects is extremely difficult. We do not know enough about the process of effective therapy to warrant assumptions about credible interpersonal interactions that would be placebos. How does one create a continuing interpersonal relationship that is presented to the client as therapy and at the same time can be demonstrated to be incapable of actually being therapy? By definition, it appears there can be no genuine and credible placebo forms of psychodynamic psychotherapy. For this reason, much of the outcome research in psychotherapy has focused on the role of patient expectancy, therapist warmth or empathy, and other supposedly non-specific aspects of therapeutic relationships as approximations to placebo effects. To the extent that many theorists suggest that these factors are central to the successful utilization of therapeutic procedures, they become active treatment effects and not placebos.

One of the supposed advantages of behaviour modification is the greater precision with which outcome studies of its effectiveness can be designed. Many forms of behaviour modification specify precise theoretical mechanisms supposedly independent of therapist characteristics which are expected to produce operationally defined symptom reduction. Within the context of this greater definitional precision, a variety of placebo possibilities present themselves.

Controlled research on placebo effects in behaviour-modification has usually focused on the issue of patient expectancy for success. The general strategy has been to present a placebo therapy to the patient with instructions that lead the patient to expect success as much as he would with the actual treatment. Careful steps are usually taken to equate time and effort of the therapist and to create conditions that are similar to the actual therapy. Finally, care is usually taken to ensure that there are no experimenter bias or demand characteristics associated with the outcome evaluation.

As careful as these procedures have been, they have not been entirely effective. Kazdin and Wilcoxon (1976) have suggested that the treatment procedures themselves, rather than any characteristics of the therapist or demands of the evaluation, may generate different expectancies for success because of their differential credibility. Lick and Bootzin (1975) wrote about the mechanisms by which such expectancy effects may work in research on systematic desensitization. Assuming that there is no magical or mystical manner by which 'expectancy' leads to therapautic success, Lick and Bootzin argued that to 'the extent to which placebo manipulations work, they must operate by mechanisms different from those traditionally proffered to explain the efficacy of (systematic desensitization)' (Lick and Bootzin, 1975, p. 926). They then suggested the following possible mechanisms. First, expecting to be cured of fear, the patient may test the expectancy by exposing himself to the feared object, thus leading to some increment in extinction of the fear. Second, expectancy changes may encourage greater attention to cues that represent improvement, leading to greater report of gain. Third, since the expectancy of improvement would be cognitively dissonant with knowledge that one still had symptoms, the dissonance may create heightened drive to continue testing reality as described above.

Biofeedback therapy, as a specific subtype of behaviour modification, seems unusually resistant to methodological shortcomings of placebo control associated with these expectancy effects. Even if a placebo therapy for biofeedback should lead to differential expectancy, it is unlikely that the mechanisms postulated by Lick and Bootzin would be applicable. First, self-reports of symptom reduction are rarely the primary criteria for success in biofeedback; quantitative changes in psychophysiological response activity are! Second, if the effect of the placebo is to cause the subject to voluntarily test the therapeutic hypothesis, it is less likely to be carried out in the visceral arena. A patient can approach a feared object in a runway more readily than he can reduce his blood pressure just to test a hypothesis. Biofeedback for tension headaches, migraine headaches, or other forms of subjective distress is theoretically presumed to work via specific measurable alterations of muscle tension, vasoconstriction, skin temperature, etc. While a placebo treatment may significantly alter the patient's subjective report of symptom reduction, it is not likely that it would similarly result in altered physiological patterns. To be sure, it is still possible that proper placebo-control research on biofeedback may be contaminated. The subject's employment of physical or cognitive mediators may be crucial to the success of biofeedback. To the extent that use of such mediators can be construed as 'work', the subject's expectancy for success may influence his motivation to work and as a result, his success with the technique. Nevertheless, my thesis is that biofeedback therapy by its very nature should be a good candidate for careful evaluation with placebo control and it is certainly better suited for such research than general psychotherapies.

In 1976 Shapiro and Surwit reviewed the biofeedback literature and arrived at the gloomy conclusion that 'there is not one well-controlled scientific study of the effectiveness of biofeedback and operant conditioning in treating a particular physiological disorder' (Shapiro and Surwit, 1976, p. 113). Two years later, Katkin *et al.* (1978) pointed out that although there have not been well-controlled experimental demonstrations of the efficacy of biofeedback therapy, the dramatic results reported with neuromuscular reeducation and with amelioration of seizure disorders were 'suggestive' of active treatment effects. Rogers and Kimball (1977), however, have adhered to stricter criteria. Discussing neuromuscular biofeedback research, they have concluded that while 'most of these studies showed fantastic results, several sources of internal invalidity ... may well account for these effects. These studies are ... inadequate in their control for the operation of even the most weak confounding variable ...' (Rogers and Kimball, 1977, p. 43).

Whether one wishes to focus on the 'fantastic' outcomes of the clinical case studies or on the inadequacy of the experimental controls employed to evaluate them, the inescapable facts are not only that no well-controlled scientific studies of the effectiveness of biofeedback therapy exist, but that there are remarkably few attempts to demonstrate such effectiveness. Researchers too frequently have omitted appropriate controls from their experiments. Even single-patient case reports rarely include appropriate baseline controls or other single-case control observations which might enhance the credibility of their conclusions (Hersen and Barlow, 1976).

SUGGESTED PLACEBO CONTROLS

After guaranteeing that control subjects are exposed to the same procedures as treatment subjects with respect to treatment milieu and instructional set, how can the biofeedback researcher provide the control subjects with credible placebo treatment? The answer is quite simple: the researcher must first possess some articulated sense of the mechanism by which the active treatment effect of biofeedback works, and then choose a form of placebo treatment which resembles it in all or most respects, but which cannot be expected to operate according to the principles of effective treatment of the biofeedback.

It has been argued (Black et al., 1977) that the effective principles by which biofeedback operates are the principles of operant reinforcement. As Katkin et al. (1978) have noted 'biofeedback ... may be seen to derive from the scientific fields of psychophysiology, learning theory, and the experimental analysis of behaviour. Specifically ... it emerged from the exciting milieu of basic research on the instrumental conditioning of autonomically mediated behaviour' (Katkin et al., 1978, p. 268). Although there has been continuing controversy over the role of so-called mediators in the operant control of autonomic responses (Crider et al., 1969; Katkin, 1971; Katkin and Murray, 1968; Katkin et al., 1969), there has been little controversy about the basic assumption that reinforcement procedures can be used to modify autonomic behaviour. Some investigators have interpreted these phenomena in traditional operant terms while others have preferred to couch their interpretations in the language of 'skills acquisition' or motor-skills learning models (Lang, 1974). Still others have focused on the role of reinforcement in modifying cognitive mediators of autonomic responses (Katkin, 1971). Regardless of the theoretical system preferred, it is widely recognized that effective control of autonomic functions requires the establishment of response-reinforcement contingencies, for it is apparent that non-contingent reinforcement of a response should have no therapeutic effect.

The simplest and most straightforward type of placebo control would seem to be false physiological feedback but I will try to convince you that it is not. It should be understood that false physiological feedback is essential to a non-contingent reinforcement paradigm, for it is likely that given veridical feedback, the subject will generate implicit reinforcements based upon knowledge of results gleaned from the feedback. Using false feedback and providing reinforcements (such as monetary rewards) that are randomly or non-contingently applied appears to be a proper control strategy. Further, one can choose to yoke control subjects with experimental ones.

As appealing and simple as this strategy appears, nevertheless it presents formidable problems. If the subject can discriminate his actual physiological response, he will soon discover the non-contingency of feedback and inquire one way or another about the discrepancy. This is a particularly acute problem in the area of skeletal-muscular feedback. Hanna et al. (1975) used false feedback of laryngeal muscle potentials in a case study of biofeedback treatment for stuttering. When they presented their patient with an interspersed control period of false feedback, he complained that the feedback instrument had gone out of adjustment. Obviously, this patient was able to discriminate veridically his laryngeal muscle tension and could perceive a discrepancy between his own internal feedback and the external feedback.

The study by Hanna *et al.* (1975) highlights the nature of a serious problem engendered by the use of false physiological feedback. If a response is discriminable false feedback will not be credible; therefore, false feedback may only be a useful control strategy for non-discriminable responses. However, Brener (1977) has argued that response-reinforcement contingencies require that reinforceable responses be discriminable. He has demonstrated that subjects are able to learn to make sensory discriminations of their visceral responses and that such discrimination enables them to gain voluntary control over those responses. This line of research and theory suggests that if a response is not discriminable, then a response-reinforcement contingency most likely cannot be established. Herein lies a paradox! If false feedback of a discriminable response is employed as a placebo control, it is likely to be detected by the subjects and thereby lose its credibility; if a non-discriminable response is employed, according to Brener (1977), it is unlikely that the contingent treatment condition will be successful. Hence, despite its inherent appeal, the use of false physiological feedback as a placebo control for biofeedback is probably inappropriate and ineffective.

Black *et al.* (1977) have argued that a major failure of research on biofeedback has been the failure to borrow from the methodological literature on instrumental learning. 'It is astonishing that so little of the theoretical and experimental armamentarium of operant conditioning has been mobilized in research on the development of control over (autonomic nervous system) and (central nervous sytem) responses' (Black *et al.*, 1977, p. 96). Black *et al.* have argued that research on biofeedback should take as a starting point the wealth of knowledge concerning the parameters of instrumental learning and should systematically study the extent to which these parameters are characteristic of treatment effects in biofeedback.

This advice is not only good research strategy, but it represents a sound conceptual base for the analysis of placebo effects. Within this paradigm, schedules of reinforcement, timing of reinforcement, magnitude of reinforcement, and other parameters of the operant experiment, can be evaluated for systematic effects on biofeedback treatment. If response to biofeedback follows the empirical laws of operant conditioning, then we can be confident that biofeedback indeed is a form of 'active treatment' and not a non-specific effect. For instance, if it could be shown that the treatment effect of biofeedback varied systematically with the schedule of reinforcement used, one could conclude that there was an active treatment effect due to operant conditioning. A variety of experimental manipulations are possible in order to gain greater insight into the nature of the active treatment effect of biofeedback.

It is generally recognized that if reinforcement is delayed, response acquisition is retarded, and that with very long delays there is no acquisition at all. For those treatment paradigms in which the feedback of physiological function is construed as a reinforcement in itself, the feedback of a physiological response can be delayed in varying degrees. Note that such a procedure, however, is isomorphic with false feedback to the extent that the subject can discriminate his physiological response. Thus it is suggested that in this situation, the subject be given specific instructions indicating that the feedback is truly of his own responses but that the apparatus will delay it in time. If contingent reinforcement is the crucial variable for a treatment effect (and not some non-specific placebo effect) the results should indicate progressively weaker treatment effects as the feedback is progressively delayed.

In a treatment paradigm in which some discrete reinforcer such as a light flash representing money is utilized, the delay-of-reinforcement procedure is more straightforward. Here presentation of the discrete reinforcer can simply be delayed. Once again, if the treatment effect is dependent on a response-reinforcement contingency, slower and less complete acquisition of visceral control should be associated with longer delays of reinforcement.

If the effects of biofeedback treatment are attributable to placebo effects, then it is likely that partial reinforcement will lead to outcomes quite similar to those achievable by continuous reinforcement. However, if the effects follow the well-established principles of reinforcement learning, then partial reinforcement schedules should result in slowed acquisition and greater resistance to extinction. With respect to biofeedback treatment, this would suggest that training with partial reinforcement should result in longer periods of symptom relief without remission or reinforcement than would be obtained with continuous reinforcement. This could be tested *in vivo*, or in a laboratory period of extinction training in which all reinforcement is discontinued. Partial reinforcement in a biofeedback paradigm can be carried out on either interval or ratio schedules.

It is well-established that ratio schedules of reinforcement result in higher rates of responding than interval schedules for simple operant conditioning. It does not follow that autonomic-response conditioning will follow similar patterns, but it does seem plausible that if the effects of biofeedback are specific to the active effect of response-reinforcement contingencies and not attributable to non-specific effects, then some clear differentiation of response acquisition should be discernible for ratio schedules of reinforcement as opposed to interval schedules.

Black *et al.* (1977) have demonstrated that in rats reinforced with lateral hypothalamic stimulation, the use of different schedules led to significantly different patterns of HR control. It is not necessary here to go into the detailed reasons for the differing results produced by two techniques of reinforcement. It is important to note, however, that the discrepancies are understandable and, more important, predictable, based on a clear analysis of the effects of differing reinforcement schedules on the pattern of response acquisition.

In order to rule out the possibility that apparent reinforcement effects are attributable to sensitization, the technique of contingency reversal, or bidirectional conditioning, has been employed. It is generally believed that if a subject can show instrumental increases and decreases in the operant level of a response as a function of differential reinforcement, then the response is not likely attributable to a placebo effect. Such considerations have guided much of Miller's early work on the instrumental modification of heart-rate response in curarized rats (Miller and DiCara, 1967). As Black *et al.* have pointed out, this bidirectional control was originally introduced in operant conditioning as a test for artifactual effects of sensitization or classical conditioning. It is essential to the proper use of this control procedure that a baseline period be employed which is characterized by random presentations of the discriminative stimuli and the reinforcers. This is necessary in order to demonstrate subsequently that both increases and decreases from baseline were actually conditioned.

CONCLUSIONS

The short history of biofeedback research is characterized by a dreary record of poorly-controlled studies. The techniques of clinical biofeedback are clearly defined and the results to date are sometimes dramatic but the confidence which can be placed in these results is low because there is little evidence bearing on the possible contribution of non-specific or placebo effects to therapeutic outcome.

False or random feedback, which appears superficially to be an appropriate placebo-control condition is probably inappropriate and is not likely to resolve the issue of specific versus non-specific treatment effects. We have suggested that the crucial distinction between an active treatment effect and a placebo effect lies in the degree to which the mechanisms underlying their effectiveness are understood. It is not legitimate to define placebo effects as those which are not understood; rather, a placebo effect is one which leads to positive outcome when knowledge of its mechanism suggests that it should not.

Biofeedback is a therapeutic tool that is well entrenched in the clinician's armamentarium. Perhaps more than any other of the clinician's tools, it is susceptible to meaningful evaluation for its specific treatment effect. The tools for this evaluation are available, and hopefully, they will soon be used.

REFERENCES

Black, A. H., Cott, A., and Pavloski, R. (1977) The operant theory approach to biofeedback training, in Schwartz, G. E., and Beatty, J. (eds.), *Biofeedback: Theory and research.* Academic Press, New York, pp. 89–128.

Brener, J. (1977) Sensory and perceptual determinants of voluntary visceral control, in Schwartz, G. E., and Beatty, J. (eds.), *Biofeedback: Theory and research.* Academic Press, New York, pp. 29–66.

Crider, A., Schwartz, G. E., and Shnidman, S. (1969) On the criteria for instrumental autonomic conditioning: A reply to Katkin and Murray. *Psychological Bulletin*, **71**, 455–461.

Hanna, R., Wilfling, F., and McNeill, B. (1975) A biofeedback treatment for stuttering. *Journal of Speech and Hearing Disorders*, **40**, 270–273.

Hersen, M., and Barlow, D. M. (1976) *Single case experimental designs.* Pergamon Press, New York.

Katkin, E. S., Fitzgerald, C. R., and Shapiro, D. (1978) Clinical applications of biofeedback: Current status and future prospects, in Pick, M. L., Leibowitz, M. W., Singer, J. E., Steinschneider, A., and Stevenson, H. W. (eds.), *Applications of basic research in psychology*. Plenum, New York, 267–292.

Katkin, E. S. (1971) *Instrumental autonomic conditioning*. General Learning Press, New York.

Katkin, E. S., and Murray, E. N. (1968) Instrumental conditioning of autonomically mediated behavior: Theoretical and methodological issues. *Psychological Bulletin*, **70**, 52–68.

Katkin, E. S., Murray, E. N., and Lachman, R. (1969) Concerning instrumental autonomic conditioning: A rejoinder. *Psychological Bulletin*, **71**, 462–466.

Kazdin, A. E., and Wilcoxon, L. A. (1976) Systematic desensitization and non-specific treatment effects: A methodological evaluation. *Psychological Bulletin*, **83**, 729–758.

Lang, P. J. (1974) Learned control of human heart rate in a computer directed environment, in Obrist, P. A., Black, A. H., Brener, J., and DiCara, L. V. (eds.), *Cardiovascular psychophysiology*. Aldine, Chicago.

Lick, J., and Bootzin, R. (1975) Expectancy factors in the treatment of fear: Methodological and theoretical issues. *Psychological Bulletin*, **82**, 917–931.

Miller, N. E., and DiCara, L. (1967) Instrumental learning of heart rate changes in curarized rats: Shaping, and specificity to discriminative stimulus. *Journal of Comparative and Physiological Psychology*, **63**, 12–19.

Rogers, T., and Kimball, W. H. (1977) *Nonspecific factors in biofeedback therapy*. Paper presented at the meetings of the Society for Psychophysiological Research, Philadelphia, Pa., October, 1977.

Shapiro, D., and Surwit, R. S. (1976) Learned control of physiological function and disease. In Leitenberg, H. (ed.), *Handbook of behavior modification and behavior therapy*. Prentice-Hall, Englewood Cliffs, New Jersey.

Stroebel, C. F., and Glueck, B. C. (1973) Biofeedback treatment in medicine and psychiatry: An ultimate placebo? *Seminars in Psychiatry*, **5**, 379–393.

Learning Theory Approaches to Psychiatry
Edited by John Boulougouris
© 1982 John Wiley & Sons Ltd

6. THE CONTEXT OF LEARNING IN BEHAVIOUR THERAPY

David Barlow

Reflecting a trend spreading quickly throughout behaviour therapy, Edward Erwin (1978), in his recent book on the scientific foundations of behaviour therapy, argues that: '... learning theory cannot now serve as an adequate foundation of behaviour therapy. It is doubtful that some of the techniques such as modelling and systematic desensitization can be logically derived from any learning theory or principle that makes no reference to mentalistic variables. Even if the derivation were possible, none of these theories or principles have been empirically confirmed and all run counter to much of the current evidence' (Erwin, 1978, p. 123). Erwin, who is actually a philosopher widely read in behaviour therapy, observes that there is no known theory or law of any kind that is of sufficient scope to serve as a foundation for behaviour therapy that has also been empirically confirmed, and that: 'We cannot even be certain that such a theory or law will ever be developed' (Erwin, 1978, p. 128). Despite this pessimism and the implication that behaviour therapy will never be anything more than a technology, Erwin does predict that an adequate theoretical base for behaviour therapy will emerge, and looks to the social learning theories of Bandura, and particularly his latest notions on self-efficacy, as a promising start.

These statements would be considered a bit extreme by most of us, but it seems important to consider Erwin's views, particularly since these views reflect a growing trend to de-emphasize the role of principles of learning in behaviour therapy.

One of the best examples of this controversy occurs in the context of aversion therapy. Aversion therapy was long thought to be based on the learning principles of classical fear conditioning, or punishment. In particular, there is one aversive procedure that has produced considerable speculation on basic mechanisms of action since this technique is carried out entirely in imagination. The procedure has been called covert sensitization by many, including its originator, Cautela (1966), although some prefer the name imaginal aversive conditioning. The basis of this procedure in clinical practice is the pairing of imagined scenes of some pleasurable but undesirable approach behaviour with additional scenes that are determined to be aversive to the patient in treatment. This technique has been most successful with cases of undesired or unwanted sexual arousal, such as exhibitionism and paedophilia (Barlow, 1978).

When used with these problems, images formed by the patient of the chain of undesired sexual behaviour are imagined in conjunction with some aversive image. In the early usage of this procedure, the aversive image was most often nausea and vomiting since these scenes seemed to be generally aversive to most people but, more recently, aversive images that are unique to each patient are determined and employed in treatment. These scenes or images are usually constructed based on the very reason the patient comes for therapy; in other words, the long-term aversive consequences. For example, when asked why they have come for treatment, most paedophiles will say that they are afraid of being arrested or losing their job or somehow embarrassing themselves and their family in front of their friends and acquaintances or possibly harming the child or children who are the object of their sexual arousal. These scenes are then incorporated into the covert sensitization process.

Before discussing the role of learning or, more precisely, conditioning, in this process, let me say that it seems this procedure is effective, at least with problems of unwanted sexual arousal. In our own clinical laboratories we have looked at the effectiveness of covert sensitization and found it to be both powerful and specific for some of these sexual problems (e.g. Brownell et al., 1977). Particularly impressive is the work of Maletzky (1980) who has recently described ten years of experience using covert sensitization with a series of 186 exhibitionists, with follow-ups extending into the ninth year. Relying on measures which include reports from both the patient and family, as well as penile plethysmography and court records, he reports no further exhibitionistic behaviour in 86% of his treated cases. It is also worth pointing out that this procedure does not seem nearly so effective with other maladaptive approach behaviours such as excessive eating, cigarette smoking, drug addiction, etc. (Barlow, 1978; Lichstein and Hung, 1980).

When this procedure was first introduced, it seemed to raise difficulties with a strict conditioning view of aversion therapy. Not only were timing variables so important in classical fear conditioning inoperative, but there were no observable stimuli (UCS) or responses (UCR) since these are presented symbolically. Although it is not clear why this procedure seems to be successful with sexual behaviour, one obvious possibility is that the over-riding cognitive bases of much sexual activity lends itself to the type of cognitive aversive intervention characterized by covert sensitization.

In any case, this procedure has been singled out, quite reasonably, by people like Wilson and O'Leary (1980) as emphasizing the significant role cognitive mediating factors play in aversion therapy, since, as both Wilson and O'Leary (1980) and Barlow (1978) have pointed out previously, covert sensitization seems basically a self-control procedure, for reasons outlined below. But if the basic principles of classical fear conditioning are not operative wherein some stimulus, even if defined in a very molar way, elicits a conditioned response, then what is the mechanism of action? Bandura (1977) argues that the effectiveness of this procedure, as well as any aversive procedure, involves using an aversive stimulus that can be easily recalled after the sessions are over, such as the sensation of a painful shock or images of nausea and vomiting. This 'stimulus' is then cognitively rehearsed, particularly when 'urges' to engage in the undesired behaviour are present. This very reasonable and commonsensical view would predict that progress would be best in those patients who rehearse the aversive images most diligently between sessions and after sessions are over. This, in turn, implies an expectancy that the procedures will be helpful and a strong motivation to change in order to maintain this behaviour of rehearsing the scene, something that obtains in most therapeutic situations.

But some of our data do not entirely support this view, no matter how reasonable it may seem. In a study published several years ago (Barlow *et al.*, 1972), we manipulated systematically the expectancies in four patients with undesired sexual arousal undergoing treatment by covert sensitization using an A–B–A–B[1] single case experimental design (Hersen and Barlow, 1976). During the first phase (A), all clients were presented with scenes of their undesired sexual behaviour and were told that imagining these scenes during deep relaxation would be therapeutic. More specifically, they were told that: 'Sexual arousal is characterized by a certain pleasurable tension which is difficult to control. This unwanted sexual arousal has been learned and we're going to get rid of the tension by substituting a relaxed response to the tension state and, in this way, eliminate your unwanted sexual arousal'. Each patient received approximately six sessions of this condition. During the second phase (B), the aversive scene was added to the scene of the unwanted sexual behaviour imagined during the first phase, along with counter-therapeutic instructions. Thus, each patient imagined the scene or situation involving the unwanted sexual behaviour paired with images of nausea and vomiting, and the instructions were designed to suggest an increase in sexual arousal: 'To obtain the best effects we're going to heighten the tension by pairing sexually arousing scenes with images of vomiting. You'll probably notice an increase in your unwanted sexual arousal and in your urges, but don't be alarmed, this is part of the treatment'. This phase also lasted approximately six sessions. The third phase (A) was a replication of the first phase where the arousing scenes only were once again presented in the context of deep relaxation, but with instructions that this would result in substantial improvement. The fourth phase (B[1]) was a return to covert sensitization, but this time with positive therapeutic instructions. What they were told was: 'You're doing well, but after reviewing your record it seems that in your case pairing the nausea and vomiting with scenes of your undesired sexual arousal is helping you the most, so we will continue with this in order to eliminate this arousal'.

Measures included the standard self-reports of sexual arousal and behaviour as well as penile circumference changes reflecting the undesired arousal, which were taken in sessions separate from the 'treatment' sessions. Debriefing indicated that three of the four subjects believed the instructions given to them during each phase (see Figure 1).

During the first phase (A), all subjects reported that they felt better and that they were practising their relaxation outside of treatment. Despite these reports, sexual arousal, as measured by penile circumference changes, remained stable. During the

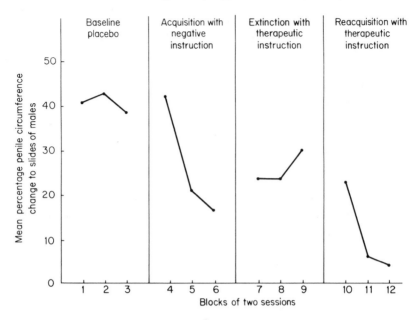

Figure 1. Mean penile circumference change to male slides for the four *S*s, expressed as a percentage of full erection. In each phase, data from the first, middle and last pair of sessions are shown. Reproduced with permission from Barlow *et al.*, *Behaviour Research and Therapy*, **10**, 411–415, 1972

next phase (B), when they received the covert sensitization, all subjects demonstrated drops in their undesired sexual arousal, with three of the four patients showing substantial drops. Despite this, three of the four patients said they were, in fact, getting worse. One noted that his erections were getting larger despite the fact they were getting smaller, and one subject developed an elaborate rationale for his worsening based on a hypothetical masochistic drive. Only one subject, the fourth, said he did not see how this could make anyone worse. When this phase was over and relaxation was once again introduced (A), all of the patients expressed considerable relief and were glad to be back in the treatment phase. One patient reported himself cured. And yet, three of the four patients showed substantial increases in their arousal. This is also reflected in the percentage change in arousal from the proceeding phase during experimental phases for each patient shown in Table 1.

It is hard to reconcile these data with a strict cognitive approach accounting for the efficacy of covert sensitization. Indeed, if the effects of covert sensitization depend on 'bringing to mind' an easily remembered aversive stimulus and rehearsing it in a self-control fashion, then there seems no reason why patients would do this during phases which they considered non-therapeutic, and yet arousal declined during these

Table 1.   Percentage change in undesired arousal during experimental phases for each S

	Covert scenes with therapeutic instruction (%)	Arousing scenes only, with therapeutic instruction (%)	Covert scenes with therapeutic instruction (%)
S1	− 51.5	+ 55.0	− 71.0
S2	− 16.5	+ 11.0	− 12.5
S3	− 3.4	+ 5.7	− 21.0
S4	− 29.5	− 3.0	− 19.5

phases. Although other investigators have found significant 'expectancy' effects during covert sensitization (Emmelkamp and Walta, 1978; Foreyt and Hagen, 1973), these investigations were in the context of problems such as smoking and excessive eating, with which covert sensitization has not been found effective (Wilson and O'Leary, 1980; Lichstein and Hung, 1980).

I cannot leave this argument entirely without bringing in some intriguing clinical observations, recognizing of course that that is not the strongest form of evidence to bring to bear on this argument. And yet, time and again, we have observed patients, particularly patients with sexual problems, report remarkable examples of what seem to be 'conditioned' responses following covert sensitization. In the early usage of this procedure, patients would come in reporting that the treatment was making them generally more nauseous in a lot of situations. Upon careful inquiry, it would be discovered that this nausea was occurring in situations where some elements of their sexual cues would be present, of which they were not aware or at least were not reporting despite having no real reason to fail to report the presence of these cues. For example, one paedophile employed in a TV repair service found himself nauseous on occasion while making repairs in certain homes. Upon examining his records and thinking back, this paedophile discovered that he was only nauseous when going into homes where there would be children who were somewhat similar to his sexual object choices and that the nausea would not occur in houses where there were only adults. A possible additional indicator of clinical success with covert sensitization in some patients is dream content. Very often during treatment, patients will come in reporting strange dreams or nightmares in which they find themselves very suddenly in the presence of their undesired object or situation followed immediately by nausea or the experience of other aversive consequences imagined during treatment. They report great surprise at this, and it does seem to correlate with a successful response to treatment.

There is little question that cognitive explanations of the ultimate success of covert sensitization, or any aversion therapy, are necessary. Any classically conditioned response in humans, if it does occur, will extinguish quickly if the patient arranges the appropriate extinction trials. One only has to remember the rather radical but futile experiments in the mid-60s where alcoholics were administered succinylcholine chloride, a respiratory paralytic, without forewarning and despite the fact that they were not motivated to give up their problem drinking (Clancy *et al.*, 1967). Conditioned responses did seem to form to this intense treatment, but almost all of the subjects were able to overcome this conditioned response within a day or so by bringing alcohol gradually closer to their lips and eventually drinking. It seems that these scenes or aversive stimuli must be rehearsed in a self-control fashion between and after sessions to insure generalization and maintenance since any 'conditioned' response would quickly extinguish once the patients left the office or laboratory where the conditioning took place and confronted the cues or discriminative stimuli associated with their undesirable behaviour.

But it seems inappropriate to throw out conditioning altogether as an important ingredient of this particular procedure, or perhaps any of our therapeutic procedures, for reasons mentioned above. Also, if aversion therapy or covert sensitization could be explained solely on mediational cognitive grounds, including rehearsing an easily remembered scene, then it would seem sufficient to construct the scene with the patient and instruct him to rehearse it repeatedly. And yet, preliminary data from our laboratories indicate that this is not effective and that the repeated pairings of the pleasurable and aversive scenes using the covert sensitization format seems necessary.

Despite difficulties in demonstrating the importance of conditioning and learning principles, or even defining these principles, one should be careful not to overlook some potentially powerful ingredients in our therapeutic procedures simply because there is little question these days that they are not sufficient to explain therapeutic effects. It is still possible that they may form, if not a necessary component, at least a very important component.

And yet, it is certain that these principles will never be sufficient in treating the complex human problems with which we are faced. In addition to theoretical explorations of the mechanisms of behaviour change in individuals, I think one of the greatest developments in years to come will be an exploration of the interaction of the social and cultural context in which any learning or behaviour change takes place. We have heard much in recent years about reciprocal determinism and the loop of causality between the behaviour of an individual and the environment in which he finds himself (Bandura, 1977); but, I am not sure that the implications of this important theoretical advance have been adequately extended to the social context. One area in which some very exciting advances are occurring concerns the social and interpersonal context of the treatment of agoraphobia. While there is no question that our behaviourally based exposure treatments, presumably operating on the basis of habituation or extinction, or possibly emotional processing, are quite effective in dealing with agoraphobia and other phobias, the interpersonal context of these treatments has been largely ignored. Recently Hafner and others (Hafner, 1976, 1977a, b; Mathews *et al.*, 1977; Chambless and Goldstein, 1980) have looked at the role the husband may play in the generation and maintenance of agoraphobia as well as its treatment. This is a particularly intriguing question since, as we know, approximately 75% of agoraphobics are women. What Hafner (1976, 1977a, b) found was that the alleviation of agoraphobia by quick acting, *in vivo* exposure methods often produced adverse effects in the husbands, resulting in increased neuroticism, occasional suicidal attempts, as well as efforts to sabotage the effects of treatment either during or after the treatment period. Recently we have begun to explore the role of the husband by actually including the husbands as cotheraptists in a twelve-session, group treatment format for agoraphobia while monitoring not only reports of the severity of phobia, rated independently by both the husband and the wife, but also objective reports of marital satisfaction (Barlow *et al.*, 1981). Treatment consisted of the usual cognitive restructuring and *in vivo* exposure accompanied and facilitated by the husband rather than the therapist. Reports of this homework as well as cognitive strategies were discussed during each of the twelve treatment sessions. Results from two couples in this initial series, illustrating these data, are shown in Figures 2 and 3.

In the first couple, a parallel relationship seems to exist in that, as phobia improves, as rated by both husband and wife, marital satisfaction also improves and the couple ends up considerably better off than before. Quite the opposite results were obtained in the second couple, however. As reports of phobia improve, once again as reported independently by husband and wife, marital satisfaction worsens, particularly on the part of the husband. It will be interesting to follow-up this couple further to determine the consequences of this deterioration, but if past clinical experience is any guide, some difficulties lie ahead for this particular couple despite the seeming success of the exposure treatment for the phobic condition.

Of course, one cannot be satisfied with examining the construct of 'marital satisfaction' in relation to agoraphobia. Questions awaiting further research include specification of the precise behaviour of the husband in generating, and maintaining, or assisting in the alleviation of the phobic response so that more efficient and effective treatments can be devised.

General systems theories, of which Bandura's (1977) reciprocal determinism is a small example, have had little impact on our therapy, in my opinion, since systems theory has not generated powerful or effective techniques for behaviour change. Nevertheless, behaviour therapy has generated powerful and effective techniques for behaviour change by most criteria (Kazdin and Wilson, 1978), and this seems to be due, in part, to the adaptation of principles of learning to clinical problems. But now that these procedures exist, we must recognize that these procedures do not operate in a social or cultural vacuum. A task for the future is a close examination of the interaction of behaviour change with the system in which it is occurring. To use a watchword of the systems theorists, one must stop thinking in a linear fashion, and some of the concepts of the systems theorists may contribute substantially to this effort (Gray *et al.*, 1969). Nevertheless, as we advance into this more complex approach to human behavioural problems therapy within a systems framework, I think it would be dangerous to lose sight of our origins and our basic principles of learning.

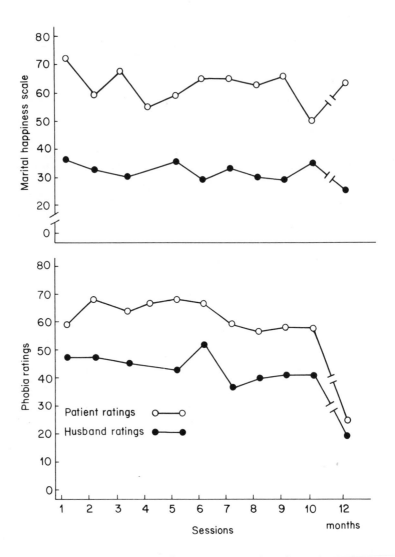

Figure 2.   Ratings of marital satisfaction and severity of phobia during treatment and at follow-up. Reproduced with permission from Barlow *et al.*, *Behavior Therapy*, in press

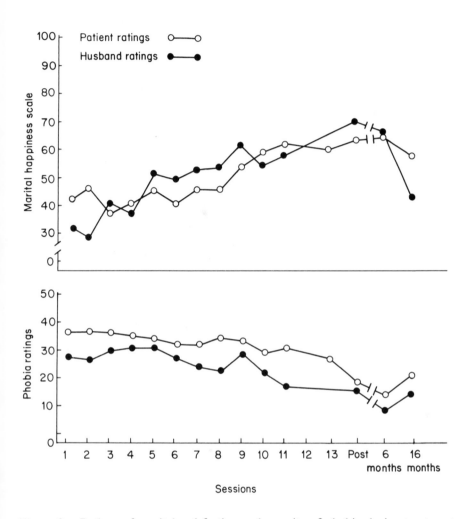

Figure 3.   Ratings of marital satisfaction and severity of phobia during treatment and at follow-up. Reproduced with permission from Barlow *et al.*, *Behavior Therapy*, in press

ACKNOWLEDGEMENT

This research was supported in part by Research Grant MH 34176 from the National Institute of Mental Health.

REFERENCES

Bandura, A. (1977) *Social learning theory*. Prentice-Hall, Englewood Cliffs, New Jersey.

Barlow, D. H. (1978) Aversive procedures, in Agras W. S. (ed.) *Behavior modification: Principles and clinical applications*, (2nd edn.) Little, Brown, Boston, pp. 86–133.

Barlow, D. H. Agras, W. S., Leitenberg, H., Callahan, E. J., and Moore, R. C. (1972) The contribution of therapeutic instructions to covert sensitization. *Behaviour Research and Therapy*, **10**, 411–415.

Barlow, D. H. Mavissakalian, M., and Hay, L. R. (1981) Couples treatment of agoraphobia: Effects on marital satisfaction. *Behaviour Research and Therapy*, (in press).

Brownell, K. D., Hayes, S. C., and Barlow, D. H. (1977) Patterns of appropriate and deviant sexual arousal: The behavioral treatment of multiple sexual deviations. *Journal of Consulting and Clinical Psychology*, **45**, 1144–1155.

Cautela, J. R. (1966) Treatment of compulsive behavior by covert sensitization. *Psychological Record*, **16**, 33–41.

Chambless, D. L., and Goldstein, A. J. (1980) Clinical treatment of agoraphobia, in Mavissakalian, M. R., and Barlow, D. H. (eds.) *Phobia: Psychological and pharmacological treatment*. Guilford Press, New York, pp. 103–144.

Clancy, J., Vanderhoof, E., and Campbell, P. (1967) Evaluation of an aversive technique as a treatment for alcoholism. *Quarterly Journal of Studies on Alcohol*, **28**, 476–485.

Emmelkamp, P. M. G., and Walta, C. (1978) Effects of therapy set on electrical aversion therapy and covert sensitization. *Behavior Therapy*, **9**, 185–189.

Erwin, E. (1978) *Behavior therapy: Scientific, philosophical, and moral foundations*. Cambridge University Press, New York.

Foreyt, J. P., and Hagen, R. L. (1973) Covert sensitization: Conditioning or suggestion? *Journal of Abnormal Psychology*, **82**, 17–23.

Gray, W., Duhl, F. J., and Rizzo, N. D. (1969) *General systems theory and psychiatry*. Little, Brown, Boston.

Hafner, R. J. (1976) Fresh symptom emergence after intensive behaviour therapy. *British Journal of Psychiatry*, **129**, 378–383.

Hafner, R. J. (1977a) The husbands of agoraphobic women: Assortative meting or pathogenic interaction? *British Journal of Psychiatry*, **130**, 233–239.

Hafner, R. J. (1977b) The husbands of agoraphobic women and their influence on treatment outcome. *British Journal of Psychiatry*, **131**, 289–294.

Hersen, M., and Barlow, D. H. (1976) *Single case experimental designs: Strategies for studying behavior change*. Pergamon, New York.

Kazdin, A. E., and Wilson, G. T. (1978) *Evaluation of behavior therapy: Issues, evidence, and research strategies*. Ballinger, Cambridge, Mass.

Lichstein, K. L., and Hung, J. H. F. (1980) Covert sensitization: An examination of covert and overt parameters. *Behavioral Engineering*, **6**, 1–18.

Maltezky, B. M. (1980) 'Assisted' covert sensitization in the treatment of exhibitionism, in Cox, D. J., and Daitzman, R. J. (eds.) *Exhibitionism: Description, assessment and treatment*. Garland Press, New York.

Mathews, A., Teasdale, J., Munby, M., Johnston, D., and Shaw, P. (1977) A home-based treatment program for agoraphobics. *Behavior Therapy*, **8**, 915–924.

Wilson, G. T., and O'Leary, K. D. (1980) *Principles of behavior therapy*. Prentice-Hall, Englewood Cliffs, New Jersey.

II. PHOBIC DISORDERS

7. IS EXPOSURE A NECESSARY AND SUFFICIENT CONDITION FOR THE TREATMENT OF AGORAPHOBIA?

Michael Gelder

In recent years, there has developed a consensus view that if agoraphobic patients are to recover they must return repeatedly to the situations which they avoid. This so-called treatment by exposure is thought to be the common theme in all the effective behavioural treatments of agoraphobia. When behaviour therapy was first introduced into Europe in the 1950s, the standard method for agoraphobia was a form of exposure treatment known as graded retraining. This gave very limited results (Meyer and Gelder, 1963) and it is a measure of the value of the research which has been carried out since then, that the latest form of exposure treatment is so much more efficient.

The research literature on exposure treatment, which is substantial, has been reviewed recently by Marks (1978) so that it is necessary only to give a summary account of the main conclusions here. The first question concerns the optimal length of exposure to the situations which the phobic patient fears and avoids. There is general agreement that prolonged and uninterrupted exposure is more effective than brief or intermittent forms (Stern and Marks, 1973; Mathews and Shaw, 1973). A period of about an hour is usually adopted in clinical practice.

The second question concerns the amount of anxiety which should be present during exposure. Many laboratory and clinical investigations now indicate that it is necessary neither to produce very low levels of anxiety by relaxation—as in desensitization treatment—nor to induce the very high levels which are part of flooding or implosion methods (Hafner and Marks, 1976; Johnston and Gath, 1973). A moderate degree of anxiety is appropriate.

The third problem is whether it is more effective to ensure that patients return to the actual situations which they avoid, than it is to require that they imagine them vividly. Marks (1978) has pointed out that many of the comparisons between real and imagined exposure are confounded because the treatments differed in other ways including the length and rapidity of exposure and the addition of relaxation or modelling. A study with volunteers which avoided these problems (Sherman, 1972) found that exposure to real situations was more effective, and Emmelkamp and Wessels (1975) reported the same with agoraphobic patients.

There is equally compelling, though less extensive, evidence that in treating agoraphobia, patients should be encouraged to take as much responsibility as possible and depend as little as possible on the therapist. In part this view derives from observations gathered by psychotherapists (Andrews, 1966). In part it originates in the observation that in most methods of behaviour therapy, improvement stops when patients cease to see their therapists (Gelder, 1977). It is possible that exposure is more effective when patients are taught how to deal with feelings of anxiety as these arise (anxiety management training), though there is no firm evidence on this point. The effects of adding biofeedback to exposure has been examined, at least with specific phobias, and has not been found to improve outcome (Nunes and Marks, 1975, 1976).

One further elaboration of exposure treatment has received considerable attention. Bandura (1971) has suggested that modelling of responses is an important agent for the treatment of phobic disorders. While this may be true for simple phobias, and especially true when the patient is a child, there is no good evidence that modelling is any more than one of several ways of encouraging patients to come into contact with the stimuli which provoke anxiety (see Marks, 1978, for a review of the evidence).

In Oxford, a form of exposure treatment has been developed which incorporates these findings in order to produce a more efficient method than those which have been available. This treatment, which we have called programmed practice, was first used by Mathews *et al.* (1977). Its essential features are:

1. Each day, for at least an hour, patients practice returning to the situations which they had previously avoided, and detailed records are kept of these journeys.
2. Except on the first occasion, the therapist does not accompany patients but acts mainly as an adviser helping them to plan what they will do without him. The therapist spends only three to five hours with the patient.
3. Each patient works with a partner (usually the husband) who joins in the planning of activities and who rewards the patient systematically for progress.
4. To ensure that they understand what they have to do, detailed written instructions are provided for both patients and partners. These written instructions take the form of a treatment manual which contains:
   (a) A convincing and reassuring explanation of agoraphobia in terms of learning of maladaptive responses.
   (b) A detailed account of graded practice, including advice on the setting of goals and sub-goals.
   (c) A description of panic management measures.
   (d) In the case of the partner, advice about the importance of encouraging the patient to be independent and about the need for frequent and immediate reinforcement of success.

We have seen that one reason for the development of this new treatment was the need to overcome the problem, encountered in all previous behavioural treatment of agoraphobia, that patients do not continue to improve after they cease to see the therapist regularly for treatment. The first test of the treatment was to see whether, in an uncontrolled study, patients would continue to improve after the end of treatment. This prediction was confirmed (Mathews *et al.*, 1977). Patients improved as much during the treatment period as they had done with the methods used before. And they went on improving after treatment ended.

The next stage was to test the method in a controlled trial in order to determine whether the results could be replicated with another group of patients and to test them against a control procedure. The latter was constructed in such a way that it contained as many as possible of the non-specific elements which are present in programmed practice. Those which appear particularly important are the effect of giving a convincing explanation of agoraphobia, the support and interest of the partner, the detailed records of progress which are made by patients and other aspects of the highly structured format of the treatment, and the great emphasis on independence and self-control. In order to include these features in the control treatment, a method was devised which was based on a 'problem-solving' approach to everyday problems. Further information about these and other points about this investigation are given by Jannoun *et al.* (1980).

In order that the two treatments should provide an equally convincing explanation of agoraphobia, patients in the control group were told that their agoraphobic symptoms were persisting because they had excessive emotional arousal. This over-arousal was explained, in turn, as the result of worry about everyday problems. Patients in the control group were told that phobias would resolve spontaneously once these life problems had been resolved, and that they need not make any special effort to practise going out; once they were calmer, they could go out just as much as they felt like doing. The structured practice in going out in programmed practice was matched, in the other treatment, by an equally structured approach to the solution of life problems: they were listed, broken down into goals and sub-goals, and tackled one by one.

The two treatments were designed to share other important non-specific therapeutic elements. Both had an instruction booklet because this presumably has a placebo effect: in the control group it provided a systematic account of the problem-solving approach. In both treatments, the therapist trained the patient in working out ways of overcoming a problem—agoraphobia in one treatment, life problems in the other. Both had equal time and attention from the therapists. Anxiolytic drugs were used as little as possible, but equally in the two groups.

Some 28 agoraphobic patients took part in the investigation and were allocated randomly to programmed practice or to the control (problem-solving) treatment, and to one or other of two therapists. Patients met the therapists five times, on each occasion in the patient's own home. This was arranged partly to ensure that in the practice group patients were going out from their own homes and partly to increase the involvement of the partner. In both treatments, patients and partner were always seen together. The first visit lasted one and a half hours and each of the others were for half an hour—in all three and a half hours spent with the therapist for treatment with two additional brief visits for follow-up.

An independent assessor rated patients before and after treatment and at the three month and six month follow-ups. Patients also filled in ratings and kept detailed daily records of their journeys from home for two-week periods before each of the assessments. Several other measures were used, but they did not conflict with the pattern of results contained in these ratings so that it is not necessary to say more about the other measures here.

The first question is whether the findings of the previous uncontrolled study were replicated. They were repeated rather closely and this is important because although scientific advance depends on replications of this kind, few have been carried out with any form of behaviour therapy. We have now compiled a manual (Figure 1) for therapists which allows others to achieve similar results after a little training (Mathews *et al.*, 1981).

Did the practice treatment, with its emphasis on exposure to phobic situations, lead to more change than the control treatment in which patients were simply told to go out when they felt ready to do so? The results indicate that it did. Figure 2 shows only the assessor's ratings but others were similar. It is noteworthy that patients who received programmed practice nearly achieved the rating of two by the three months

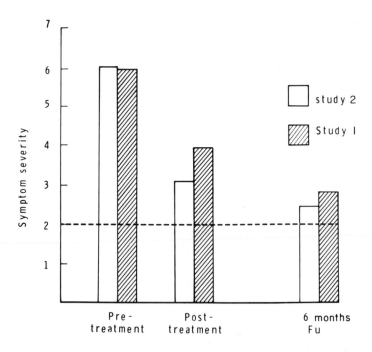

Figure 1.   Assessors ratings of symptom severity: study 1 and study 2

follow-up, for this rating indicates that symptoms are mild and not associated with any avoidance or impaired social functioning. So far, then, the results support the hypothesis that improvement was related to the treatment component which is specific to programmed practice, that is exposure to the feared situations.

However, there was a further stage in the analysis. We have seen that two therapists took part in the trial, each treating an equal number of patients from the two treatment groups. When the results of these two therapists were compared, the results were unexpected. They obtained almost identical results with programmed practice, but with problem-solving their results were different. One therapist obtained results with the two treatments which were not significantly different, while the other therapist obtained results which were significantly less good with the control treatment than with programmed practice.

What can explain this interesting and unexpected finding? The first possibility and that which is most relevant to the theme of this paper, is that the first therapist was breaking the rules of the problem-solving treatment and encouraging patients to practice going out when she should not have been doing this. However, when the number of hours spent away from home by patients in each treatment group were analysed separately for each therapist, there was no evidence that this was

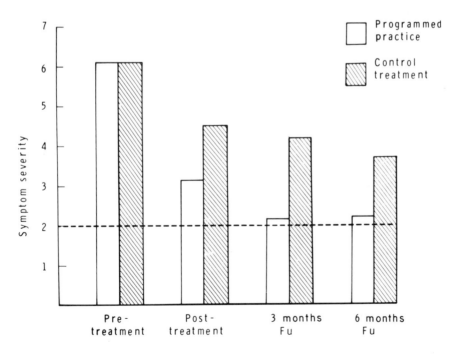

Figure 2. Assessors ratings of symptom severity (0–8 scale), before and after treatment

happening. Moreover, neither control group was going out significantly more than at the beginning of treatment. Thus the results do not support this explanation and we are left to look for another.

When ratings of general anxiety were examined in the same way, it was found that the patients of the therapist who obtained better results with problem-solving were rated as having shown a greater reduction in general anxiety than those of the other therapist. It is possible that this greater reduction in general anxiety in the more improved patients was instrumental in bringing about their greater improvement. Unfortunately, we are not sure *why* anxiety fell more in this group. To understand these findings, it is necessary to remember that phobic severity ratings encompass both anxiety and avoidance. The results indicate that although the programmed practice groups were carrying out their daily tasks, their experience of going about everyday journeys was no different to that of the more successful subgroup of those who received the control procedure. Moreover, by the end of the follow-up, the programmed practice and control groups were no longer significantly different in the amount they went out—and their over-all ratings of phobic symptoms were similar as well.

How do these findings relate to the question posed in the title of this chapter? Is exposure a sufficient condition for the treatment of phobic states? We can only give a qualified answer to this question. As carried out in programmed practice, exposure is sufficient, but in this treatment it is not used alone but combined both with anxiety management techniques and with considerable efforts to replace attitudes of helplessness with those of self-efficacy. If we remember the limited results which were obtained years ago with graded retraining, in which exposure treatment was used without these two additional measures, then we would be unwise to conclude that exposure is a sufficient condition. One way of interpreting this is to suppose that the behavioural procedure of exposure to avoided situations does not, by itself, produce the cognitive changes which are required for complete recovery; and that the additional measures are necessary to induce these cognitive changes.

If exposure treatment is not a sufficient condition, is it a necessary one? Before we can answer this, we have to say what we mean by exposure. The term is only useful when it also means more than the ordinary commonsense efforts which patients would make if they were given no special advice. As a technical term it therefore implies a systematic and determined effort to re-enter situations which have been avoided. If this definition is used, then our results suggest that exposure may not be a necessary condition, for we believe that one control subgroup made only commonsense attempts to go out, and yet improved. This finding must be replicated before it can be accepted with confidence but until this has been done it does at least suggest that there may be more than one way of bringing about change in phobias. One possibility is that the final common path for improvement of phobias is exposure to feared situations, but that this can be a rather gradual and unsystematic process. If this is true, we can go on to observe that there may be more than one way of bringing this exposure about—by vigorous exposure as in programmed practice, or by making patients generally less anxious and more self-confident. Another more speculative view would be that the final common path is cognitive change—fewer fearful expectations and a stronger feeling of being in control—and that these can be brought about in ways which do not require specific re-exposure. This view suggests further investigation of the value of the structured format of programmed practice and its components of anxiety management. We can conclude that although programmed practice now offers an efficient and effective treatment for agoraphobia, there are still plenty of interesting problems left for the research worker who wants to understand more about the mechanisms by which behaviour can be made to change. Until these are solved we can only give a qualified answer to the question which we set out to answer.

ACKNOWLEDGEMENTS

The programme of research in Oxford has been carried out in collaboration with Andrew Matthews and Derek Johnston; and the most recent investigation with Pepe Catalan, Leila Jannoun, and Mary Munby. It was supported by the Medical Research Council.

REFERENCES

Andrews, J. D. W. (1966) Psychotherapy of phobias. *Psychological Bulletin*, **66**, 455–480.

Bandura, A. (1971) Psychotherapy based on modelling principles, in Bergin, A. E., and Garfield, S. L. (eds.) *Handbook of Psychotherapy and Behaviour Change*. (1st edn) Wiley, New York, 653–708.

Emmelkamp, P. M. G., and Wessels, H. (1975) Flooding in imagination versus flooding *in vivo*. A comparison with agoraphobics. *Behaviour, Research and Therapy*, **13**, 7–13.

Gelder, M. G. (1977) Factors which limit improvement after treatment of agoraphobia, in Boulougouris, J., and Rabavilas, A. (eds.) *The Treatment of Phobic and Obsessive Compulsive Disorders*. Pergamon, Oxford, 7–12.

Hafner, J., and Marks, I. M. (1976) Exposure *in vivo* in agoraphobics: the contributions of diazepam, group exposure, and anxiety evocation. *Psychological Medicine*, **6**, 71–88.

Jannoun, L., Munby, M., Catalan, J., and Gelder, M. G. (1980) A home-based treatment for agoraphobia: replication and controlled evaluation. *Behaviour Therapy*, **11**, 294–305.

Johnston, D. W., and Gath, D. H. (1973) Arousal levels and attribution effects on diazepam assisted flooding. *British Journal of Psychiatry*, **123**, 463–466.

Marks, I. M. (1978) Behavioural psychotherapy of adult neurosis, in Garfield, S. L., and Bergin, A. E. (eds.) *Handbook of Psychotherapy and Behaviour Change*. (2nd edn.) John Wiley, New York, Ch. 13, 493–548.

Mathews, A. M., and Shaw, P. M. (1973) Emotional arousal and persuasion effects in flooding. *Behaviour, Research and Therapy*, **11**, 587–598.

Mathews, A. M., Teasdale, J., Munby, M., Johnston, D. W., and Shaw, P. M. (1977) A home-based treatment programme for agoraphobia. *Behavior Therapy*, **8**, 915–924.

Mathews, A. M., Gelder, M. G., and Johnston, D. W. (1981) *Agoraphobia: Nature and Treatment*. Guilford Press, New York.

Meyer, V., and Gelder, M. G. (1963) Behaviour therapy and phobic disorders. *British Journal of Psychiatry*, **109**, 19–28.

Nunes, J., and Marks, I. M. (1975) Feedback of true heart rate during exposure *in vivo.* *Archives of General Psychiatry*, **32,** 933–936.

Nunes, J., and Marks, I. M. (1976) Feedback of true heart rate during exposure *in vivo.* Partial replication with methodological improvement. *Archives of General Psychiatry*, **33,** 1346–1347.

Sherman, A. R. (1972) Real life exposure as a primary therapeutic factor in desensitisation treatment of fear. *Journal of Abnormal Psychology*, **79,** 19–26.

Stern, R. S., and Marks, I. M. (1973) A comparison of brief and prolonged flooding in agoraphobics. *Archives of General Psychiatry*, **28,** 210–214.

Learning Theory Approaches to Psychiatry
Edited by John Boulougouris
© 1982 John Wiley & Sons Ltd

8. FACILITATION AND INHIBITION OF FUNCTIONAL CS EXPOSURE IN THE TREATMENT OF PHOBIAS

Thomas Borkovec

Research on anxiety-related disorders over the past few years has documented to a fairly conclusive extent that exposure to feared stimuli is the *sine qua non* of effective treatment (cf. Mavissakalian and Barlow, 1980). Those behavioural techniques experimentally demonstrated to be effective with phobias or obsessive–compulsive disorders, for example, desensitization, *in vivo* and imaginal flooding, participant modelling, and reinforced practice, share the common ingredient of repeated or prolonged exposure to anxiety-related material. This conclusion, drawn by many researchers in the field on the basis of a steadily growing and impressive body of investigations, is highly significant and establishes a solid basis for future research directions aimed at the ultimate resolution of anxiety-related disorders. Those further directions follow rather clearly from that conclusion, in terms of the unanswered questions that surround its statement.

First, although repeated or prolonged exposure is the effective procedural ingredient, we are aware of neither the process of its influence nor the mechanisms whereby its therapeutic effectiveness is established. So few data have been collected from the various, crucial response domains (cognitive, physiological, and behavioural) during the actual conduct of treatment that we lack an adequate description of the process of change. With regard to mechanism, extinction is often invoked, yet this principle is in the strictest sense only a description of a procedure or a description of the effects of such a procedure and not an explanation.

Second, the numerous forms of exposure treatment are not equally effective with all disorders. *In vivo* flooding, for example, is superior to imaginal desensitization in the treatment of most obsessive–compulsive and phobic problems. Although exposure appears to be a necessary condition, its effectiveness depends on other aspects surrounding the procedure (e.g. duration of exposure, presence or absence of relaxation, performance feedback, and models). Furthermore, the facilitative role of these auxiliary aspects of procedure most likely relate differentially to (1) the type of disorder being treated; (2) the characteristics of the clients receiving the treatment, and (3) the site of effect for the procedure in terms of the response domain maximally influenced. Future research will, therefore, no doubt attempt to identify what procedures adjunctive to the basic exposure operations will facilitate extinction for which kinds of people and by what mechanisms.

Thirdly, while the efficacy of current techniques is beyond dispute, we still have a long way to go in technique development before we can be confident that the vast majority of anxiety-related disorders can be efficiently eliminated with long-lasting effects. Many clients remain uninfluenced by even our most powerful treatment procedures, and we must identify the client characteristics that contribute to this lack of effect.

In an evolutionary sense, the extinction process is of obvious significance for survival: fear behaviour to realistically life-threatening conditions maintains the species. Stimuli which may elicit initial fear but are not truly dangerous should, with repeated exposure, lose their ability to evoke useless and maladaptive responses. Furthermore, extinction may be viewed along a rather fundamental continuum of repeated exposure effects which include habituation and monotonous stimulation. Specifically, fear responses decline with repetition of the feared stimulus in the absence of punishment, orienting responses decline with repetition of a neutral stimulus once the organism adjusts to its presence and significance (Sokolov, 1963), and sleep is the natural consequence to a continuation of repeated non-signal stimuli (Bohlin, 1971). Thus, the decline of responsiveness with repetition is a common descriptive statement across the entire range of stimuli from emotional to non-emotional and probably reflects a common, fundamental principle of behaviour.

If that process is so fundamental, then the primary question for anxiety researchers may not be why extinction takes place, although that question is certainly heuristic and its pursuit will no doubt lead to elucidation of the neurological and biochemical events underlying this basic phenomenon. Rather, what is intriguing is why extinction fails to take place in that subset of people who develop neurotic problems. This failure is seen in two forms: the lack of complete success in eliminating neurotic disorders by current techniques and the maintenance of anxiety for some period of time prior to effective treatment despite frequent exposure experienced by the client in his/her everyday circumstances. The latter failure raises the question of why phobics ever become and remain phobic, given that extinction is a natural, fundamental, and evolutionary adaptive process for most people.

Our own interest has been in this question and our primary focus has been on what the person does to prevent exposure and thereby prevent extinction process. We assume that repeated exposure will naturally lead to extinction but that whether or not functional exposure takes place is dependent on the extent to which the client actually allows that exposure to occur. So we are concerned with what the client does to prevent the occurrence of CS exposure, despite objective presentation of those fear stimuli in the environment or during therapy, and what auxiliary conditions may facilitate the functional impact of the basic repeated exposure procedure.

Mowrer (1947) suggested three decades ago that instrumental avoidance of an aversively conditioned CS complex serves to maintain anxiety. While subsequent work has questioned the relevance of this two-stage model of fear for human neurosis, it remains a useful paradigm, especially if extrapolations can be made which take into account some characteristics of human behaviour.

We assume that what phobics do to mitigate CS exposure is to avoid the relevant fear stimuli, and this avoidance, though sometimes at the overt behavioural level, most often takes place in cognitive, perceptual, and attentional processes. The hypothesized common denominator for these processes in the case of the phobic is that they reduce awareness of or attention to the phobic stimuli and thereby preclude functional CS exposure and hence extinction. The variety of cognitive styles and the content of those styles may reflect enormous individual differences based on learning history, but their function is posited to be the same: avoidance of the feared stimuli.

A second assumption is that two major classes of fear-relevant stimuli must be considered: external, environmental fear cues and internal cues which include both thoughts and images as well as physiological responses. We often forget that the CR is part of the CS complex, and consequently exposure to those response-produced stimuli is theoretically of some importance.

Let me briefly summarize some of the research findings from our laboratory which form the basis for these assumptions.

For several years, we have assessed individual differences in the extent to which phobics report awareness of physiological responses when they are anxious. We know from several laboratories that autonomic perception reports do not correlate strongly with actual physiological activity; they are usually orthogonal. However, in every study in which this subject characteristic was factored into the design, it significantly interacted with exposure manipulations to determine whether incubation or extinction occurred. For example, Stone and Borkovec (1975) in a one-session study found evidence for an incubation effect under exposure conditions of moderate duration, whereas brief as well as prolonged exposure produced fear reductions. Importantly, this paradoxical enhancement of fear occurred only among those subjects who reported a high awareness of physiological cues. Furthermore, we have evidence that fearful subjects who are accurate in their reports of physiological cues (i.e. there is concordance between those reports and their actual heart rate responses to the phobic stimulus) display extinction with repeated *in vivo* exposure, whereas inaccurate or discordant subjects show fear maintenance (Borkovec, 1973). These outcomes fit well conceptually with the findings of Lang *et al.* (1970) of greater process and outcome improvement among subjects showing agreement between self-reported fear and heart rate during desensitization. Moreover, the role of awareness of fear response components during repeated exposure has been recently stressed in Lang's (1977) information processing account of phobic imagery and its emphasis on the importance of incorporating response propositions into the phobic scene descriptions.

Many years ago, we found that explicitly instructed imaginal avoidance maintains fear. Snake phobic subjects received either desensitization, implosive therapy, or an avoidance response placebo treatment. Subjects in the latter condition visualized the same phobic scenes as in desensitization, were subsequently imploded until they signalled anxiety, at which time they then visualised a standard avoidance response. Tonic heart rate remained high throughout four sessions of treatment and outcome improvement was negligible, relative to the changes occurring in the two therapy conditions. Thus, cognitive avoidance of feared stimuli can result in fear maintenance, despite repeated exposure. Grayson and Borkovec (1978) conducted a one-session replication of the imaginal avoidance response condition on speech phobic subjects and compared it with a group which visualized mastering the situation and a group which imagined not coping, i.e. experienced intense physiological reactions. Three phobic images were each presented three consecutive times. Reported fear was least for the mastery condition, with less evidence of fear reduction for the avoidance condition and some evidence for incubation among the not-coping condition.

Research therefore supports the idea that extinction of feared stimuli will take place to the extent that the client attends to or is aware of relevant fear stimuli during the repeated exposure. This includes response-produced physiological cues, the presentation of which may initially contribute to a paradoxical enhancement of fear under brief exposure conditions. If this is the case, then we may ask what conditions might increase such awareness and reduce our tendency to avoid the feared material, and thus facilitate otherwise naturally occurring extinction processes. Active, forceful techniques such as flooding, implosive therapy, and response prevention exemplify one avenue. The client's likelihood of engaging in avoidance is reduced under the persistent and direct exposure procedures employed, and these strategies appear to be effective in accomplishing this task, although a good deal of client discomfort occurs as a consequence. Traditional psychotherapy has long taught us the alternative approach: establishment of an accepting, comfortable therapeutic atmosphere and therapist encouragement of exploration of feared material. The same phenomenon can be observed in our own lives, when intimate and open friendships characterized by trust and lack of fear of criticism allow discussion of fears and concerns that we otherwise would not verbalize, perhaps even to ourselves. We would therefore expect that conditions which maximize comfort during exposure, or promise relief as a consequence of attending to stimuli that are painful and therefore customarily avoided, should mitigate avoidance and facilitate extinction. Our past research has suggested that two commonly manipulated variables in behavioural fear research, relaxation and expectancy, may function in precisely this way.

Our first evidence that expectancy may facilitate functional CS exposure came in Grayson's study mentioned above (Grayson and Borkovec, 1978). In addition to the mastery, coping, and not-coping conditions, speech anxious subjects were randomly assigned to either positive, therapeutic expectancy, or neutral expectancy, i.e. the groups differed in terms of whether they were told that repeated imagination of speech-related scenes would produce a reduction in their fear of public speaking. Subjects given therapeutic instructions showed greater reported fear upon initial presentation of each scene, and greater decline with repetition relative to neutral expectancy subjects. Heart rate showed a similar pattern: greater initial reactivity and greater decline within image presentations and across repetitions for positive expectancy subjects. It appears that subjects are more willing to expose themselves to fear content if there are motivating conditions to do so (e.g. 'I'll lessen my fear in the future if I confront the feared situation') than if such motives are not induced. Evidence of this greater functional exposure derives from the greater subjective and cardiovascular impact of initial presentations, and the customary decline with repetition to be expected from effective repeated exposure.

This study involved only a single session and outcome effects were unexpected in such a context. Borkovec and Sides (1979) recently reported a four-session desensitization study with speech anxious subjects, which included the expectancy manipulation and thus provided an opportunity to replicate Grayson's effect.

Three groups of subjects received equivalent durations of imaginal exposure to a phobic hierarchy. One group was progressively relaxed during exposure and followed customary desensitization procedure. The remaining two groups imagined the scenes without relaxation. One of these latter groups was relaxed during the last half of the session subsequent to a half-hour of hierarchy exposure; thus both components of desensitization were present, though non-contiguously. Half of the subjects in each group were given therapeutically-oriented, positive expectancy instructions, whereas the other half received neutral instructions. Desensitization produced evidence of functional CS exposure. The initial presentation of the first image resulted in greater heart rate response, greater decline over images, and routine decline with repetition of each image. The other two conditions gave less evidence of systematic reaction or change. Expectancy produced the same influence as we found in Grayson's one-session study, but only during the first session. And during the first session, the expectancy effect was clear only in the two conditions without relaxation. Presence of relaxation over-rode the more tenuous expectancy influence. Our conclusion from these data is that both relaxation and expectancy can serve as motivating conditions for facilitating functional CS exposure and thus extinction, hypothetically via their capacity to reduce cognitive avoidance. It appears that the expectancy effect is short-lived, however, and cannot maintain this role without some other supporting devices during subsequent sessions. The presence of relaxation significantly related to subjective outcome improvement, whereas expectancy had no effect on post-test anxiety.

Obviously, we require better methods for assessing attention in these studies in order to test the hypothesized role of awareness and avoidance in phobic process. Our current and future work will utilize beat-by-beat analysis of cardiovascular responses to phobic stimuli, hopefully allowing for the discrimination of defensive responses, thought to reflect rejection of environmental inputs, from orienting responses associated with attention to the inputs. Secondly, if phobics do avoid fear material perceptually or attentionally, then tasks involving recognition of ambiguous phobic and non-phobic stimuli should demonstrate for phobic individuals longer reaction times and a shift in cardiovascular activity from orienting to defensive responses as the clarity of the feared stimulus is increased. Finally, while some interesting hypotheses about fear process have emerged from this research, it is clear that replication needs to be conducted on a wider range of fear problems, including of course clinically severe phobias. We are currently developing single-subject procedures with clinical patients which will provide opportunities to assess cognitive, physiological, and behavioural reactions to both imaginal and *in vivo* presentations of phobic stimuli prior to and after therapy, as well as physiological and self-report measures during the conduct of exposure treatment.

Although our research has focused predominantly on imaginal exposure procedures and the role of relaxation in those techniques, we are not thereby arguing that these treatment modalities are somehow more important or effective than other modes. On the contrary, the literature clearly indicates that *in vivo* exposure is the current treatment of choice, while relaxation is not a necessary aspect of exposure therapy. As mentioned earlier, however, we know very little about the mechanisms involved in the exposure treatment of phobia, subject characteristics will no doubt interact with various modes of presenting exposure procedures, and each variation will have perhaps differential impact on different response systems. It may be, for example, that imaginal techniques may be useful for eliminating fear mediated by thoughts and images in anticipation and in reaction to environmental exposures, whereas *in vivo* exposures are principally effective for eliminating overt avoidance and fear reactions directly elicited by environmental stimuli.

Any exposure treatment can provide the experimental context for a pursuit of laws of behaviour, as long as we go deeply into that context in a systematic and programmatic way. As a basic researcher, my concern is with the identification and description of phobic process and of the mechanisms involved in the maintenance and reduction of that process. The need for relaxation, the potency of imaginal procedures, the role of expectancy, these issues are important not for their applied implication but for their role as independent variables in the experimental elucidation of the nature of phobias.

I would like to conclude with an example of the use of relaxation in the experimental analysis of a different problem, that of general anxiety. While learning theory and research have been applied to the problem of specific phobia for several decades, far less attention has been paid to diffuse fear, although major developments have occurred in agoraphobia, a possibly related disorder. In my clinical experience and that of several colleagues we have often found that the application of relaxation results in a paradoxical increase in anxiety among generally anxious clients. Typically, they report initial feelings of relaxation followed by a growing sense of vague apprehension during the middle portion of the session. These experiences are often sufficiently unpleasant to result in aborting the training. Something about the relaxation experience apparently causes anxiety. It would appear that some internal stimulus conditions serve as the elicitors, either physiological sensations or cognitive events. The possibility of relaxation-elicited fear has already been demonstrated in the animal laboratory by Denny (1976) who found that incipient relaxation cues, if associated with aversive events, can retard usual fear extinction processes. This phenomenon provides a ready explanation perhaps for some subtypes of diffuse anxiety. External elicitors cannot be identified because the major CS for the occurrence of fear is internal. Since that internal condition is relaxation, the client remains at high level of anxious arousal. From our previous work on the role of internal cues in fear, we would expect that exposure to such internal cues may lead initially to an increase in fear, followed by fear reduction if exposure is sufficiently repeated or prolonged.

We recently began a series of investigations on general anxiety in the normal population, and the results have thus far supported the occurrence of relaxation-induced anxiety. In one study, generally anxious subjects were randomly assigned to one of three groups: (1) progressive relaxation training which combines tension and release of muscle groups with instructions to focus on the resultant physiological sensations, (2) no-treatment, and (3) a group which received relaxing images in place of physiological attention-focusing (Borkovec and Hennings, 1978). Progressive relaxation resulted in an increase in daily tension level reports over the four-week duration of the study, whereas the pleasant imagery group showed improvements significantly greater than progressive relaxation and no-treatment. Apparently, brief relaxation which draws the subjects' attention to physiological cues can lead to an incubation of fear, while techniques which induce pleasant feelings via imagery circumvent exposure to relaxation-induced stimuli. More recently, Rebecca Grayson (1978) found increases in frontal EMG among high anxious subjects treated in one session with relaxation techniques involving attention to physiological cues, whereas low anxious subjects showed no change or declines in EMG.

The most recent study of this type was just completed by Heide (1980). Chronically anxious clients ranging in age from 18 years to 61 years were given one session of progressive relaxation and one session of mantra meditation in counterbalanced order. Multivariate analysis of physiological and subjective report measures indicated that progressive relaxation was superior to the meditation procedure overall. However, 36% of the former group and 43% of the latter reported greater anxiety at the end of the session than before the session began. Furthermore, increases in skin conductance measures, heart rate, respiration rate, and frontal EMG occurred among 10–47% of the subjects, depending on the index used. We are currently conducting regression analyses in order to predict the occurrence of this phenomenon on the basis of a variety of subject characteristic measures obtained prior to the treatment sessions. It appears, however, that exposure to relaxation sensations can result in anxiety and, secondly, that shutting down customary cognitive activity via a mantra device can also be fear-eliciting. Numerous hypotheses could be suggested to account for this phenomenon, e.g. fear of physiological events in general, fear of relaxation sensations in particular as Denny's theory suggests, fear of loss of control elicited by the shut-down of cognition usually used to maintain the client's world view. Our future work will attempt to isolate the mechanisms involved, but it is quite likely that there is more than one subtype of generally anxious clients for whom the phenomenon is characteristic.

In conclusion, little explicit attention has been paid to the role of awareness of both external and internal fear cues in the origins, maintenance, and reduction of anxiety-related disorders. As methods from information processing and related areas of research are applied to these problems, we may perhaps reach a better understanding of the mechanisms of these disorders and develop techniques sufficient for the effective and efficient elimination of neurosis.

REFERENCES

Bohlin, G. (1971) Monotonous stimulus, sleep onset, and habituation of the orienting reaction. *Electroencephalography and Clinical Neurophysiology*, **31**, 593–601.

Borkovec, T. D. (1973) The role of expectancy and physiological feedback in fear research: A review with special reference to subject characteristics. *Behavior Therapy*, **4**, 491–505.

Borkovec, T. D., and Hennings, B. L. (1978) The role of physiological attention-focussing in the relaxation treatment of sleep disturbance, general tension, and specific stress reaction. *Behaviour Research and Therapy*, **16**, 7–19.

Borkovec, T. D., and Sides, J. K. (1979) The contribution of relaxation and expectancy to fear reduction via graded imaginal exposure. *Behaviour Research and Therapy*, **17**, 529–540.

Denny, M. R. (1976) Post-aversive relief and relaxation and their implications for behavior therapy. *Journal of Behavior Therapy and Experimental Psychiatry*, **7**, 315–322.

Grayson, J. B., and Borkovec, T. D. (1978) The effects of expectancy and imaginal response to phobic stimuli on fear reduction. *Cognitive Therapy and Research*, **2**, 11–24.

Grayson, R. (1978) *Effects of relaxation with vs. without muscle tension-release on muscle activity of low and high anxious subjects*. Unpublished honours thesis, University of Iowa.

Heide, F. J. (1980) *Relaxation-induced anxiety: A psychophysiological investigation*. Unpublished doctoral dissertation, The Pennsylvania State University.

Lang, P. J. (1977) Imagery in therapy: An information processing analysis of fear. *Behavior Therapy*, **8**, 862–886.

Lang, P. J., Melamed, B. G., and Hart, J. (1970) A psychophysiological analysis of fear modification using an automated desensitization procedure. *Journal of Abnormal Psychology*, **76**, 220–234.

Mavissakalian, M. R., and Barlow, D. H. (1980) *Phobia: Psychological and pharmacological treatment*. Guilford Press, New York.

Mowrer, O. H. (1947) On the dual nature of learning—re-interpretation of 'conditioning' and 'problem-solving.' *Harvard Educational Review*, **17**, 102–148.

Sokolov, Y. N. (1963) *Perception and the conditioned reflex*. Pergamon Press, Oxford.

Stone, N. M., and Borkovec, T. D. (1975) The paradoxical effect of brief CS exposure on analogue phobic subjects. *Behaviour Research and Therapy*, **13**, 51–54.

Learning Theory Approaches to Psychiatry
Edited by John Boulougouris
© 1982 John Wiley & Sons Ltd

9. THE ROLE OF THE FAMILY MEMBER IN THE SUPPORTED EXPOSURE APPROACH TO THE TREATMENT OF PHOBIAS

Jerilyn Ross

The supported exposure approach to the treatment of phobias combines short-term group counselling with individual therapy (DuPont, 1979). The latter is administered by a phobia therapist, either a mental health worker or a former phobic who has been trained to guide phobics into real life anxiety-producing situations while teaching specific anxiety-reducing techniques. The phobia therapist helps phobics set achievable goals and take the necessary steps to be able to enter into and to remain in the phobic situation long enough to see that the feared reactions (i.e. going crazy, having a heart attack, fainting) will not occur and that intense anxiety levels will diminish (Ross, 1980).

During the group session the leader, generally a psychiatrist or some other mental health professional, spends the first 20 minutes of the 90-minute session focusing on one particular aspect of the phobic process, i.e. dealing with anticipatory anxiety, goal setting, handling setbacks. During the remainder of the session phobics discuss their accomplishments and disappointments of the previous week, with emphasis placed on learning to feel good about achievements, no matter how small. Family members or other support people are encouraged to attend and to participate in the group session.

The degree of support phobics receive from family members affects the outcome of treatment. In a recent study of 18 agoraphobic married women, Milton and Hafner (1979) found that overcoming phobias often causes severe marital problems because neurotic symptoms can cement a marriage and when the mental health of one spouse improves, the relationship between the partners sometimes deteriorates. Hardy, however, observed over 100 couples in his agoraphobic treatment programme and concludes that regardless of personality type, spouses who participate in treatment are less resistant and more willing to accept change in their mate and also to make changes in themselves (Hardy, 1979).

103

The supported exposure approach emphasizes the seriousness of phobic fear, focusing on it as a real, severe experience which is not imagined by phobics and is not the same as the 'fears' of non-phobics. This enables both phobics and family members to see the phobia as a real handicap rather than something to feel guilty or make judgements about. Thus it becomes a shared problem which can be overcome by hard work and which can produce pride rather than shame. Prior to treatment, family members often try to cover up and excuse or to blame phobics for the disability and inconvenience. During treatment they are taught to encourage, support, and celebrate. When neurotic patterns get in the way, these too are approached as practical problems to be overcome with the support of the group. Family members are not made to feel guilty for undermining the phobics' progress. Instead, they are made aware of their behaviour and shown how to be supportive by changing it. By including non-phobic family members in the group sessions, the non-supportive family members learn how to become supportive and the supportive, but ineffective family members learn how to become effective.

HELPING THE SUPPORT PERSON BECOME EFFECTIVE

Feelings of shame and embarrassment about asking for help and/or appearing foolish often lead phobics to hide their anxiety and, yet, at the same time, to expect others who are close to them to be 'sensitive enough' to realize they are experiencing difficulties. Rarely does phobic anxiety manifest itself externally (Zane, 1978); therefore, phobics have to be taught to take responsibility for letting others know when they are having a problem. Rather than passively waiting for a family member to initiate support and then becoming angry and disappointed when it is not given, phobics are taught to say: 'I am feeling phobic and would like your help'. It is important for phobics to be able to tell the person who is helping them exactly what is helpful and what is not. At times phobics need to be held or talked to; at other times they want to do the holding or talking and, sometimes, they want to be left alone. The support person has to understand that these inconsistencies in needs have to do with the nature of the phobia and should not take them as a personal rejection.

Much of the anxiety phobics experience has to do with their fear of loss of control (Marks, 1978). To be able to enter into the phobic situation, phobics need to feel in control of themselves and of their environment, including everyone around them. The more control phobics feel they have over the situation, the less they feel trapped and thus less anxious. The non-phobic might ask: 'What would you like me to do to help you feel more comfortable?' and not act offended or put out by the reply. Phobics are taught to tell the family member exactly what would be reassuring, even if the request is irrational. For example, a young woman who was afraid of going into high buildings for fear she would lose control and jump out the window asked her boyfriend to reassure her that if she did lose control, he would knock her out so she would not be in any danger of hurting herself. They both knew how absurd this request really was, but having this reassurance enabled the woman to go up to the high floor and remain there long enough to see that her feared reactions would not happen.

Phobics always need an 'out' and it is helpful to decide with the family member what this will be prior to entering the phobic situation. For example, if a person is hesitant to go into a crowded theatre for fear of panicking and having to leave, the family member might suggest: 'Let's get tickets and go with the understanding that if you wish to leave at any time you may, even if it is in the middle of the performance, and that I will leave with you'. This is difficult to say because the support person is often afraid that this kind of leniency perpetuates the phobia. However, just knowing that a way out is an option enables phobics to enter phobic situations. Once they are confident that they are not trapped and trust that their family member would leave without being critical, it becomes easier to enter into the feared situation.

As phobics begin to get better, they experience concern about what will be expected of them now that they have demonstrated that they can do the things which they were previously unable to do (Weekes, 1976). It is helpful for them to express this concern to the person helping them. For example, the phobic might ask the helper: 'Since I did the shopping today, will you expect me to do it all the time?', 'If I drive to the party tonight, will I have to drive home?', or 'If I go up in the elevator, can I walk down the steps if I want to?'. The family member should assure the phobic that there are no additional expectations and should help the phobic to focus on the present. When phobics do not feel the pressure to perform, they are more likely to enter into and remain in feared situations.

Family members often cannot understand that phobics may be able to do something with a stranger, their phobia therapist, and yet not be able to do the same thing with them. This increases the family member's frustration and doubt regarding the intensity of the phobic's fear, which causes the phobic to become more defensive and withdrawn. The thought that there is an expectation to perform and that there will be judgement, raises the phobic's anxiety level, which perpetuates phobic thinking and decreases willingness to confront the phobic situation. It is common for phobics to do the same task several times with little or no discomfort and then suddenly feel paralysed and unable to proceed. The phobia therapist understands this and explains it to the phobic. The family member, however, sees it as an indication of the phobic's inadequacy. In order to be helpful, the supportive family member must convince the phobic that support will be provided irrespective of whether the phobic completes the task.

THE ROLE OF THE FAMILY MEMBER DURING THE PRACTICE SESSION

The supportive exposure approach involves encouraging phobics to take two steps forward while allowing them to take one step back. The family member often asks: 'When am I being supportive and when am I being too pushy?'. This fine line is illustrated in the following hypothetical conversation between a phobic person (PP) and an effective, supportive family member (FM). The phobic's goal in this practice session was to drive two blocks.

PP: I really don't think I can do it today.

FM: How about if we just get into the car and you turn on the ignition?

PP: OK, but that's all I can do, I'm too scared.

PP and FM enter car. PP turns on ignition.

FM: How about just driving to the end of the block?

PP: No way.

FM: Can you just go to the end of the driveway?

PP: I don't know. I feel so silly. OK, I'll try.

PP drives to end of driveway.

FM: Good. Now, let's go to the end of the first house.

PP: I can't. What if I panic and lose control?

FM: Stay in the present. Are you panicking now? Notice that your hands are firmly on the wheel, that your feet are where they belong and that you are functioning perfectly well. Remember, your feelings are frightening, but not dangerous. You won't do anything you don't want to do.

PP: What if I get on to the road and want to run out of the car?

FM: That's OK. I'll take over the wheel.

PP takes deep breath and drives to end of the first house.

PP: I can't believe I did it, but it's really no big deal.

FM: It's terrific and it is a big deal. A few minutes ago you didn't think you could drive at all and now you have driven. Let's go three more houses and then you can turn back.

PP: I can't do that.

FM: You didn't think you could get this far and you did. You're OK.

PP: OK, three more houses and that's all. Keep talking to me.

PP goes three more houses.

PP: I'm scared. I want to go back. You promised.

FM: OK. We'll go back. Try to count to 20 first. (Allow anxiety to pass)

PP counts to 20 and feels better. Still wants to go back. Does so and is immediately encouraged to move forward again. This time, goes directly to third house and is surprised at feeling comfortable. Looks carefully at FM for any indication of impatience. Sees look of support and encouragement. Continues on to end of block and, then, end of second block. Repeats whole process several times before ending session.

The phobic person was able to achieve the goal and a sense of satisfaction because:

1. Specific goals were set.
2. Goals were approached one step at a time.
3. 'Outs' were clearly defined and permitted.
4. Achievements were reinforced.
5. Progress, no matter how small, was acknowledged.
6. Patience and commitment were evident on the part of the family member, with no evaluative judgement.

7. Reality was tested.
8. Phobic let family member know exactly what would be helpful.
9. Phobic was encouraged to remain in situation until high anxiety level diminished, but was not forced or humiliated into staying.
10. Phobic was not made to feel weak and/or helpless.

Phobics have a hard time feeling good about their achievements, especially since phobias often develop in areas they previously had no difficulty with. A business executive who developed a fear of elevators, for example, found it difficult to get excited about going three floors in an elevator when he used to ride up and down all day without even thinking about it. It is critical, however, that every step forward, no matter how small, be acknowledged as progress and looked at relative to the beginning of treatment. The businessman's wife was instructed to help him realize that two weeks ago he was unable to go into the elevator at all and today he was able to go three floors. He was encouraged to feel proud of himself and not to feel inhibited about sharing his accomplishment with his wife and other family members.

CHANGING ROLES AS A RESULT OF TREATMENT

Prior to treatment phobics are preoccupied with phobic thinking, often to the extent that other emotions are ignored. Much of the phobics' time and energy is spent trying to avoid and manipulate people and situations which they fear will trigger a panic attack. Because they feel guilty for being so demanding and dependent, phobics often feel that they have no right to assert themselves in other areas. Thus some emotional needs are ignored and the resulting frustration further perpetuates anxiety and adds strain to their relationships. During treatment, phobics are taught to increase their awareness of their emotional needs and to become more assertive. As this change takes place, the non-phobic family member often feels less needed, more threatened and confused, and sometimes attempts to keep the phobic passive and dependent.

Case I

Mrs A had been unable to leave her house for nine years without her husband, who appeared to be very supportive. Following her eighth week of treatment and two successful shopping trips with her therapist, Mrs A decided to attempt to go shopping on her own. She was so excited about being alone and not feeling panicky that she stayed in the store much longer than she had anticipated. When her husband came home from work and did not find her at home, as usual, he became frantic. When Mrs A arrived home 20 minutes later, expecting Mr A to be as excited as she was about her accomplishment, she was, instead, confronted with anger and hostility.

Comment Clearly, Mr A was frightened that something may have happened to his wife. During the following week's group session, it was suggested to Mrs A that a phone call to her husband, explaining where she was and that she might be late, could have easily avoided the unpleasant situation and might have resulted in his sharing her excitement. It was further suggested that Mrs A needs to recognize the potential effects the changes she is going through may have on her husband and the importance of her being aware of his feelings, as well as expecting him to be aware of hers.

Case II

Mrs B had been housebound for three years and after nine weeks of treatment excitedly announced to her husband that she accepted a part-time job as a typist. Mr B was outraged and threatened to 'cut the wires' in her car if she tried to go to work. He argued that her 'role' was to be at home and take care of him and their children and not to be out working around other men all day.

Comment During her next individual therapy session, it became obvious that part of Mr B's reaction had to do with the way Mrs B told him about her acceptance of a job. Rather than being honest and saying that now that she was able to go out, she did not want to stay in the house all day and that she felt the need to do something for herself, Mrs B told her husband that she was taking a job because they needed the money. Mr B, a very proud and traditional man, interpreted this as her telling him he was not a good provider. This brought up many of his own insecurities and resulted in his feeling embarrassed and humiliated by the thought of his wife having to work. Once both partners became aware of this miscommunication, the issue was resolved. They decided to put the money Mrs B earns into a special bank account and use it to take a vacation, something they had been unable to do previously because of her agoraphobia.

RELATING TO CHILDREN

Case III

Mrs C had been phobic for 42 years relative to elevators, driving, and thunderstorms. During a conversation with her eldest child, now 37 years old, Mrs C mentioned that she was being treated for her phobias. Her daughter said she was shocked to find out her mother had suffered all these years. She had no idea. She then recalled being a youngster in grade school and feeling angry and neglected when there would be a rain storm and all the mothers except hers would come to pick up their children. Mrs C always seemed to be waiting for some delivery, having something on the stove, or having a headache. Her daughter remembers thinking that if her mother really loved her, she would not make her walk home in the rain. Mrs C, on the other hand, talked about the pain and guilt she felt when her fear of thunderstorms and driving was so great that even the thought of her loved ones walking home in the rain could not get her to confront her fears. She was too humiliated and embarrassed to ask her neighbours to pick up her children because, as is typical of phobics, Mrs C was sure that if she did ask they would think she was crazy.

Comment Mrs C was afraid to tell her children the truth for fear they might 'catch' the fear or that they might make fun of her. She now realizes that the negative effect which this had on her relationship with her children was much more devastating than if she had told them the truth. Telling children of their parents' fears and how it affects their behaviour may be less damaging than allowing the children to think they are unloved.

In relating to children, phobics are encouraged to explain the fear in terms of fears children can relate to, i.e. fear of the dark, of the 'bogey man', or strange noises. It should be explained that grown-ups are also sometimes afraid of things which they really do not have to be afraid of, and that things may be frightening to some people and not to others. This often helps children to understand their parents' fear, and to feel better about their own fears. Children are often much more accepting and tolerant than adults imagine and can be helpful to phobics if they are included in the practice sessions. Children can help set goals, participate in reality testing exercises and help phobics find simple, manageable taks that can help the phobics to focus on the present.

CONCLUSION

The amount of progress phobics make during treatment is often dependent upon the degree of support they receive from their spouse or other family members. By including these support people in the group sessions and teaching them how to become supportive, they are able to share the excitement of progress rather than feel left out and confused by the changes that may occur in their relationships as a result of treatment. It is important for phobics to realize that, even if family members are supportive, it is difficult for non-phobics to recognize when phobics are experiencing panic or for them to fully understand what phobic fear is like. Therefore, phobics are taught to take responsibility for letting others know when they are feeling phobic so they can get the help, support, and encouragement that is so vital to their progress.

REFERENCES

DuPont, R. L. (1979) *Profile of a phobia treatment program: first year results.* Paper presented at the 132nd annual meeting of the American Psychiatric Association. Chicago, Illinois, May 18, 1979.

Hardy, A. B. (1979) *The role of the spouse in the treatment of the agoraphobic patient.* Paper presented at the 132nd annual meeting of the American Psychiatric Association. Chicago, Illinois, May 18, 1979.

Marks, I. (1978) *Living with fear.* McGraw Hill, New York.

Milton, F., and Hafner, J. (1979) The outcome of behaviour therapy for agoraphobia in relation to marital adjustment. *Archives of General Psychiatry*, **36**, 807–811.

Ross, J. (1980) *The use of former phobics in the treatment of phobias. American Journal of Psychiatry*, **137**, 715–717.

Weekes, C. (1976) *Agoraphobia*. Hawthorn Books, Inc., New York.

Zane, M. D. (1978) Contextual analysis and treatment of phobic behavior as it changes. *American Journal of Psychotherapy*, **32**, 338–350.

Learning Theory Approaches to Psychiatry
Edited by John Boulougouris
© 1982 John Wiley & Sons Ltd

10. SELF-CONTROL PSYCHOTHERAPY WITH AND WITHOUT EXPOSURE TO ANXIETY

Athanassios Constantopoulos, Philip Snaith, Yvonne Jardine, and Nick Bolsover

The importance of self-control in behavioural psychotherapy has been emphasized during the last decade by an increasing number of authors (Bandura, 1969; Kanfer, 1970; Meichenbaum, 1975; Gelder, 1979). A significantly better short-term outcome for phobic patients whose treatment programme provides for exposure to phobic situations, along with critical examination of the three main variables involved (level of anxiety, duration of exposure, and its form) has been described by various authors (Crowe *et al.*, 1972; Mathews and Shaw, 1973; Johnston and Gath, 1973; Stern and Marks, 1973; Emmelkamp and Wessels, 1975; Mathews *et al.*, 1976). Examination of some contradictions between these results paved the way to the realization of the more important role of systematic homework by the administration of instruction manuals (Mathews *et al.*, 1977). These points have been reviewed recently by Gelder (1979) along with other strategies employed between sessions with the therapist.

The present project is an attempt to invetigate some of the factors involved in the above findings, during therapy of phobic patients with the programme of '*anxiety control training*' i.e. hypnotic sessions followed by autohypnotic practice as had been modified by Snaith (1981). The null hypotheses tested in the programme of 'anxiety control training' were as follows:

1. Exposure to focalized anxiety does not improve the short-term outcome.
2. Improvement in the severity of focalized anxiety is not dependent upon improvement in generalized anxiety.
3. There is no difference in the degree of improvement in generalized anxiety between patients exposed to anxiety during the programme.

Phobic patients complying with the inclusion criteria of the study were stratified into three groups, according to the duration of their main area of phobic symptomatology, as follows: (1) short, i.e. less than three years; (2) medium, i.e. between three and eight years; and (3) long, i.e. more than eight years.

Having been allotted to one of the three groups, patients were randomly allocated to either 'A' therapy group, i.e. introduction of anxiety scenes during sessions and encouragement of active countering anxiety situations between sessions or 'C' therapy group, i.e. instructed in techniques of coping with anxiety but without actual exposure to anxiety by the therapist or encouragement to enter anxiety provoking situations in everyday life.

Following allocation to their particular therapy group, the patients were then given explanations of the treatment programme and handed the appropriate manual for their autohypnotic exercises at home. The manuals for group 'A' and 'C' differed in that instructions for exposure to anxiety between sessions were present in the 'A' manual but absent in the 'C' manual.

The patients completed the IDA scale (Snaith et al., 1978), the FSS scale (Snaith, 1968), and the PQRST (Mulhall, 1976) in which items relating to the main phobia, an unrelated phobia, and the generalized anxiety were included. The therapist and an independent assessor completed phobic anxiety-rating scales similar to those of Watson and Marks (1971). For anxiety and avoidance, five-point rating scales were completed. Following completion of the rating scales at the commencement of treatment, the therapist informed the patients that, although he will personally supervise the treatment, they will be seen by an independent assessor again some time after the tenth treatment session. The IDA and PQRST scales were completed again before commencement of the sixth session.

At the end of the tenth session, the therapist made a global assessment of the patient's application to the programme and progress. Between two and four weeks after the tenth therapy sessions, the patients were interviewed by the independent assessor, who was supplied with the items that were written on the PQRST and the main and unrelated phobias on the phobia scales, but was given no other information about the patients and was instructed not to ask patients about details of their treatment, which may have betrayed which group they were in. The assessors asked the patients during this interview to complete all ratings (IDA, FSS, PQRST) and they themselves completed the phobic anxiety rating scales and 'global' rating was made to assess the general progress of treatment.

The patients were taken through the first hypnosis session and at the end of this session were instructed to start practising the exercises as outlined in the manual at home. Treatment sessions, ten in all, were generally conducted weekly and each session lasted 20–30 minutes.

RESULTS

A total of twelve patients have completed the trial up to now, comprising five males and seven females. The age range was between 20 and 45 years. Table 1 shows the random allocation of the patients into 'A' and 'C' treatment groups according to the duration of their main area of phobic symptomatology. Group 'A' consisted of four male and two female patients. Group 'C' consisted of one male and five female

Table 1. Patients allocation according to symptom duration

	Short <3 years	Medium 3–8 years	Long >8 years
Group 'A'	2	1	3
Group 'C'	2	2	2

patients. Table 2 shows the outcome measured between groups 'A and 'C' (Mann–Whitney U-test). As can be seen, there are no significant differences between

Table 2. Results derived from Mann–Whitney U-test between groups

	U	p	
Focalized anxiety (assessor's ratings)	12	0.197	NS
Focalized anxiety (self-rated PQRST)	17	0.469	NS
Focalized avoidance (assessor's ratings)	16	0.409	NS
Assessor's global rating of outcome	15	0.350	NS
Generalized anxiety (self-rated IDA)	17	0.469	NS

groups 'A' and 'C' as far as short-term outcome is concerned and therefore null hypotheses (1) and (3) are upheld. As far as the relationship of improvement in focalized to improvement in generalized anxiety is concerned, the Spearman rank-correlation coefficient was $+0.7$ $p<0.05$ and therefore null hypothesis number (2) is refuted. Table 3 shows the outcome in relation to the duration of the main area of phobic symptomatology. The division into three groups of outcome is produced by a

Table 3. Treatment outcome in relation to symptom duration

	Symptom free	Marked improvement	Some improvement	No improvement
Short <3 years	2	2	0	0
Medium 3–8 years	2	0	1	0
Long >8 years	1	2	2	0

combination of the improvement shown in assessor's ratings and self-rated (PQRST) focalized anxiety.

DISCUSSION

As is evident from the results, exposure to focalized anxiety during the 'anxiety control training' programme, does not improve the short-term outcome. This result is not in keeping with the recent literature and although it remains to be seen whether any differences emerge during a longer follow-up of the patients participating in this study, some speculations regarding these preliminary results would be appropriate at this point.

Our research was primarily addressed to the problems of whether phobic patients need to learn a general coping strategy or whether they need to learn to cope with specific situations. These preliminary results seem to support the former notion and possible explanations could be as follows. Exposure to anxiety is of much less importance in a programme such as the 'anxiety control training' which:

1. Primarily is 'sold' to the patient as a 'package deal' emphasizing the patient's active participation and rigorous practice at home, much more than the rather traditional assumption of the all important time spent with the therapist. It is made clear to the patient from the beginning of the process that he is primarily responsible for failure or success and that the therapist's role is a secondary one as teacher or trainer who will help the patient with the initial steps of acquiring the coping skill.

2. Incorporates an instruction manual given to the patient containing clear explanations about the nature of anxiety, his role in the whole programme, and the homework he is expected to do between sessions without the therapist. The manual, as well as the detailed discussion of it between patient and therapist, is a powerful instrument in helping to shift the emphasis from the therapist to the patient as the protagonist in the whole process of treatment.

   Both explanations enhance the chances of the notion of self-mastery (Frank, 1974, 1976) or self-efficacy' (Bandura, 1977), that is central to all psychotherapeutic systems, and in recent times much attention has been drawn to these two aspects (Gelder, 1979).

3. As an integral part to the whole approach, instills in the patient the expectation of anxiety relief by a coping mechanism which will help the patient to overcome anxiety. This last factor would be in agreement with Bandura's theories of self-efficacy and self-referent thought.

   Bandura makes three points about self-referent thought which bear on this aspect of skill development. Firstly, having a coping skill in itself contributes to a sense of personal efficacy. Secondly, potential threats largely activate fear through cognitive self-arousal and thus the belief that one can control anxiety will attentuate self-arousal. Thirdly, avoidance of situations results in a failure to develop coping strategies. Having learnt a coping process people are in a position to further develop skills in previously avoided situations.

If these three explanations are used for a synthesis, then it seems that a cognitive–behavioural model could emerge to explain the results. In this kind of model the over-riding factor for improvement would be of a successful 'selling' of a 'theory' (package deal) to the patient, which the patient gradually adopts as his own and comes to use and experiment with in every day life situations. It might also be possible that the stronger his belief and acceptance of the 'theory', the higher his motivation and chances of tackling successfully previously feared and avoided situations, which in turn reinforces his belief in the 'theory' and sustains his motivation to test out his theory in more and new situations.

In the context of such a model the instruction manual assumes a different role to the one traditionally assigned to it. Instead of merely being an instrument of clarification and understanding, it becomes an instrument derived from and in line with the 'theory'. In other words the facts of the instruction manual fit the 'theory' that the patient has been developing and therefore reinforce further belief and acceptance of the 'theory', along with increased and more successful use of the manual as a logical extension of such a theory.

REFERENCES

Bandura, A. (1969) *Principles of Behaviour Modification*, Holt, Rinehart and Winston, London.

Bandura, A. (1976) Self reinforcement: Theoretical and methodological considerations. *Behaviourism*, **4**, 135–155.

Bandura, A. (1977) Self-efficacy: Toward a inifying theory of behavioural change. *Psychological Review*, **84**, 191–215.

Crowe, M. J., Marks, I. M., Agras, W. S., and Leitenberg, H. (1972) Time limited desensitization, implosion, and shaping for phobic patients. *Behaviour Research and Therapy*, **10**, 319–328.

Emmelkamp, P. M. G., and Wessels, H. (1975) Flooding in imagination vs. flooding *in vivo*: a comparison with agoraphobics. *Behaviour Research and Therapy*, **13**, 7–15.

Frank, J. D. (1974) Psychotherapy: The restoration of morale. *American Journal of Psychiatry*, **131**, 271–274.

Frank, J. D. (1977) The two faces of psychotherapy. *Journal of Nervous and Mental Disease*, **164**, 3–7.

Gelder, M. G. (1979) Behaviour therapy as self-control, in: Gaind, R. N., and Hudson, B. L. (eds.). *Current Themes in Psychiatry*, Macmillan Press, London, pp. 165–177.

Johnston, D. W., and Gath, D. (1973) Arousal levels and attribution effects in diazepam assisted flooding. *British Journal of Psychiatry*, **123**, 463–466.

Kanfer, F. H. (1970) Self regulation: research, issues and speculation, in Nouringer, C., and Michael, J. L. (eds.). *Behaviour Modification in Clinical Psychology* Appleton-Crofts, New York, pp. 178–220.

Mathews, A. M., and Shaw, P. M. (1973) Emotional arousal and persuasion effects in flooding. *Behaviour Research and Therapy*, **11**, 587–598.

Mathews, A. M., Johnston, D. W., Lancashire, M., Munby, M., Shaw, P. M., and Gelder, M. G. (1976) Imaginal flooding and exposure to real phobic situations: treatment outcome with agoraphobic patients. *British Journal of Psychiatry*, **129**, 362–371.

Mathews, A. M., Teasdale, J., Munby, M., Johnston, D. W., and Shaw, P. M. (1977) A home based treatment programme for agoraphobia. *Behaviour Therapy*, **8**, 915–924.

Meichenbaum, D. (1975) A self instruction approach to stress management, in Sarason, I., and Spielberger, C. D. (eds.) *Stress and Anxiety*, Wiley, New York, Vol. 2, pp. 227–263.

Mulhall, D. J. (1976) Systematic self-assessment by PQRST. *Psychological Medicine*, **6**, 591–597.

Snaith, R. P. (1966) Phobia scales. *British Journal of Psychiatry*, **112**, 309–319.

Snaith, R. P. (1981) *Clinical Neurosis*, Oxford University Press, Ch. 7, pp. 208–227.

Snaith, R. P., Constantopoulos, A. A., Jardine, M. Y., and McCuffin, P. (1978) A clinical scale for the self-assessment of irritability. *British Journal of Psychiatry*, **132**, 164–171.

Stern, R. S., and Marks, I. M. (1973) Brief and prolonged flooding: a comparison in agoraphobic patients. *Archives of General Psychiatry*, **128**, 270–276.

Watson, J. P., and Marks, I. M. (1971) Relevant and irrelevant fear in flooding. *Behaviour Research and Therapy*, **2**, 275–293.

III. OBSESSIVE–COMPULSIVE DISORDERS

Learning Theory Approaches to Psychiatry
Edited by John Boulougouris
© 1982 John Wiley & Sons Ltd

11. RECENT DEVELOPMENTS IN THE BEHAVIOURAL TREATMENT OF OBSESSIVE–COMPULSIVE DISORDERS

Paul Emmelkamp

Recent research into the treatment of phobic (Emmelkamp, 1979) and obsessive–compulsive patients (Emmelkamp, 1982) has stressed the importance of exposure *in vivo*. Although treatments for obsessive–compulsives have become known as participant modelling or flooding, exposure *in vivo* plus response prevention seem to be the essential components of these procedures. There is no evidence that modelling enhances the effects of exposure *in vivo* (Boersma *et al.*, 1976; Emmelkamp, 1981).

Self-controlled exposure *in vivo* has been found to be about equally effective as therapist-controlled exposure *in vivo* in the treatment of obsessive–compulsive patients (Emmelkamp and Kraanen, 1977). With self-controlled exposure *in vivo* the patient has to practise therapeutic tasks in his natural environment. At the beginning of therapy a hierarchy is constructed of stimuli that trigger obsessive–compulsive behaviour. Each session the patient receives homework assignments consisting of items from the hierarchy. The patient has to expose himself to situations which provoke rituals and he is not allowed to carry out his rituals. This form of treatment can best be conceived as gradual exposure *in vivo* plus self-imposed response prevention.

The advantages of self-controlled exposure are obvious. Firstly, the role of the therapist is reduced to that of a teacher. The therapist teaches the patient how he can carry out his own treatment. Secondly, treatment needs less therapist time. Thirdly, treatment is conducted in the natural environment of the patient, thus preventing problems of generalization. Finally, there is some clinical evidence indicating that checkers may profit more from self-controlled exposure than from therapist-controlled exposure.

Family members of obsessive–compulsives are often involved in the rituals of these patients. Family members have often to carry out the same washing rituals as the patient in order to reduce patient's anxiety. In the case of checking rituals, patients can avoid the provocation of some of their rituals by trusting their partner to do these activities. Finally, some patients seek constantly reassurance from their partners by questions as: 'Are you sure I didn't cause an accident', 'Is that non-poisonous', or 'Did you wash your hands'. Partners often accommodate to the wishes of the patients and hence reinforce the obsessive–compulsive behaviour.

We were interested whether the involvement of the partner in the treatment would enhance the effectiveness of treatment by self-controlled exposure *in vivo*. Therefore, we designed a study in which two conditions were compared: (1) self-controlled exposure by the patient alone and (2) self-controlled exposure with assistance of the patient's partner. Twelve obsessive–compulsives who had a relationship of at least one year's duration were randomly assigned across these two conditions.

In the *patient alone* condition, treatment consisted of self-controlled exposure *in vivo* along the lines of Emmelkamp and Kraanen (1977). Each session patients received instructions from the therapist how he should practise therapeutic tasks in his natural environment. In this condition the patient's partner was neither involved in the discussions with the therapist, nor in the execution of the homework assignments. Family members were instructed to be absent during the practice hours.

In the *couple condition* the partner had to accompany the patient each treatment session. After the rationale was explained to the couple, the patient received instructions for self-controlled exposure. He had to carry out his homework assignments with his partner present. The task of the partner was to encourage the patient and to have him confront the stimuli which distressed him until the patient gets used to them. As in the patient alone condition, the patient was not allowed to perform his rituals. Treatment in both conditions consisted of four information sessions and ten treatment sessions. There was no practising of the tasks during treatment sessions.

Although the study is not yet finished, the preliminary data may be of some interest. Both treatment conditions led to significant improvements, but the couple condition proved to be superior to the individual condition on some of the measures. Figure 1 presents the data of both groups on the self-rating anxiety scale (Watson and Marks, 1971). In this figure the data for the main obsessive–compulsive problem and the other obsessive–compulsive problems have been combined. Clearly, the couple condition led to more improvement than the condition in which the patient was individually treated.

These preliminary data suggest that the involvement of family members in the treatment of obsessive–compulsives may be profitable. Remarkably, even in cases with clear marital discord the partner could be involved in the treatment without disrupting treatment progress. It is interesting to note that both treatments led to a slight increase in satisfaction with the marital relationship as measured by the Maudsley Marital Questionnaire.

So far the role of the partner; let us now turn to the cognitive ruminations of obsessive–compulsive patients. Although obsessive–compulsive rituals are often triggered by cognitive ruminations there is no evidence that cognitive modification

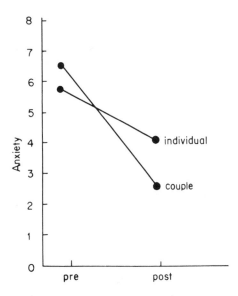

Figure 1.   Self-rating of anxiety (main and other obsessive–compulsive problems combined)

procedures along the lines of Meichenbaum (1975) are of any value with this population. Emmelkamp *et al.* (1980) compared (1) exposure *in vivo* and (2) self-instructional training followed by exposure *in vivo* and found no differences in effectiveness between both conditions. Thus, self-instructional training seem to be of little value in the treatment of obsessive–compulsive patients. Similar meagre results were found with agoraphobics (Emmelkamp *et al.*, 1978).

A better way to change the cognitive ruminations of obsessive–compulsives may be prolonged exposure in imagination (Emmelkamp and Kwee, 1977). With this approach patients are exposed to their obsessions for a prolonged period and are not allowed to perform neutralizing activities. We suppose that prolonged exposure to the obsessions without cognitive escape and avoidance behaviour may lead to habituation. Figure 2 shows the subjective anxiety ratings of one selected patient. Clearly, a curvilinear pattern of subjective anxiety occurs during each treatment session, demonstrating that prolonged exposure to the obsessions indeed leads to habituation.

After having established the usefulness of this approach in a pilot study (Emmelkamp and Kwee, 1977), we were next interested in whether the effects of this procedure were due to habituation to the obsessions or whether the effects could be accounted for by habituation to fear in general. Therefore, two variants of prolonged exposure in imagination were compared in a crossover design. Thus, each patient was used as his own control. Six obsessional patients who evidenced no clear rituals served as subjects in this study. Treatment in each phase of the experiment consisted

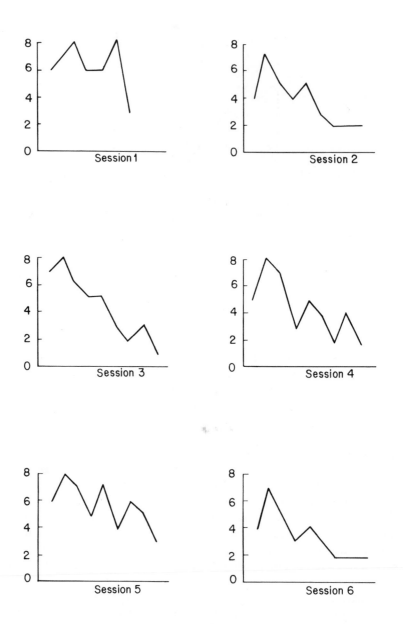

Figure 2. Subjective anxiety ratings of one patient during treatment by prolonged exposure in imagination to obsessions. Reproduced with permission from Emmelkamp, *Obsessions and Compulsions: Recent Advances in Behavioral Analysis and Therapy*, Springer, 1982

of six sessions of one hour's duration. Relevant exposure consisted of prolonged exposure to the obsessions; irrelevant exposure consisted of exposure to themes as being burnt to death, being strangled, being devoured by a tiger etc.

Total treatment led to significant improvements on the Leyton Obsessional Inventory (Cooper, 1970) and to significant reductions in the frequency of the obsessions. Comparing relevant versus irrelevant exposure it was found that relevant exposure was clearly superior to irrelevant exposure. With several patients, irrelevant exposure even led to an increase of the frequency of the obsessions and to an enhancement of the distress experienced. The results of this study suggest that the essential component of this treatment involves habituation to obsessions instead of to fear in general. However, it should be remembered that only a small number of obsessional patients were involved in this study. It needs hardly to be argued that the data presented here need to be replicated before more definitive conclusions can be drawn about the effectiveness and the essential therapeutic components of prolonged exposure in imagination.

The subsequent discussion is directed mainly at the clinical management of obsessive–compulsive patients. Behavioural research into the treatment of obsessive–compulsives almost exclusively has dealt with the effectiveness of various exposure procedures and with parameters influencing its outcome. Since behavioural theories about the development and the maintenance of obsessive–compulsive disorders have relied heavily on the anxiety reduction hypothesis, it is not surprising that most of the behavioural research in this area has focused on exposure procedures. Although the procedures have been found to be effective, it needs to be stressed that not all patients can be helped by these methods. In addition, some of the patients who derive benefit from treatment by exposure need additional treatment for related problems. Thus exposure procedures are not the panacea for obsessive–compulsive patients.

In a number of obsessive–compulsives the rituals seem to serve another function. Clinical observations suggest that obsessive–compulsive patients are often social-anxious and unassertive. In some of these cases the obsessive–compulsive problems might serve the function of avoiding people. In such cases exposure and response prevention procedures alone are usually of limited value and need to be supplemented by other therapeutic interventions. Let me illustrate this point by a case report.

The patient was a 32-years-old unmarried woman with extensive obsessive–compulsive problems. As she defined the problem, she was afraid of contaminating other people and therefore she had to avoid contact with people. She had no relationships, lived socially isolated, and no one was allowed to visit her home. At the start of the treatment the patient denied any problems in social relationships. In her view, the lack of acquaintances and friends were not the cause but the result of her obsessive–compulsive problems. Initially, treatment was directed to her obsessive–compulsive problems by means of gradual exposure *in vivo* plus response prevention. Although rather slow, treatment along these lines progressed as long as direct contact with people was avoided. At that time the therapist discussed with her the possibility that the rituals could serve the function of avoiding people because of her anxiety in social situations. Although the patient was reluctant to accept such a definition of her problem, she finally agreed upon treatment of these problems by assertive training. During the course of the assertive training the patient became aware that her obsessive–compulsive problems were enhanced when she was criticized or when she did not know how to deal with social situations. After having become more assertive, the patient succeeded on her own initiative in shaking hands with people, joining social clubs, taking dancing lessons, and inviting people to her own home without feeling urges to execute compulsive rituals. The evidence in this case is incomplete because delayed effects of the exposure *in vivo* phase cannot be ruled out. Although this case report contains no more than a slight hint of a link between social anxiety and obsessive–compulsive problems, the value of assertive training in overcoming obsessional problems deserves further study.

In the light of our often successful treatment of obsessive–compulsive patients with assertive training after preceding exposure *in vivo* treatment, it became a matter of interest to know whether assertive training on its own would lead to a reduction of the obsessive–compulsive problems. Another case study may yield some information that is of direct bearing on the present question. The patient was a young man in his early 20s with obsessive–compulsive checking as his main problem. He worked as a motor mechanic and his work took at least four times as long as his colleagues. On the ground of a functional analysis it was hypothesized that his compulsive checking was caused by his social anxiety and unassertiveness.

To test the putative relationship between unassertiveness and obsessive–compulsive problems the patient was treated with assertive training. After a baseline period of three weeks twelve sessions of assertive training followed. Treatment was conducted twice weekly. The patient had to report on social situations in which he was unassertive or he felt uneasy. These situations were discussed and a more adequate handling of these situations was trained through modelling by the therapist and through behaviour rehearsal. After each session the patient received homework assignments in order to use his newly acquired skills in his daily live. These homework assignments followed a hierarchy and involved situations as looking at people, starting a conversation with strangers, inviting people home, refusing requests etc. After this phase of treatment baseline conditions were reintroduced and then treatment focused directly on his obsessive–compulsive problems by means of self-controlled exposure *in vivo*. Exposure *in vivo* lasted for six weeks (seven sessions). Then the post-test was applied.

Figure 3 represents the patient's daily ratings of his obsessive–compulsive problems during the course of treatment. Clearly, assertive training led to a clinically significant reduction of his obsessive–compulsive problems. During the second phase of treatment (exposure *in vivo*) the improvement continues. Figure 4 presents the data at pre-test, intermediate test, and post-test for the self-rating of fear, the

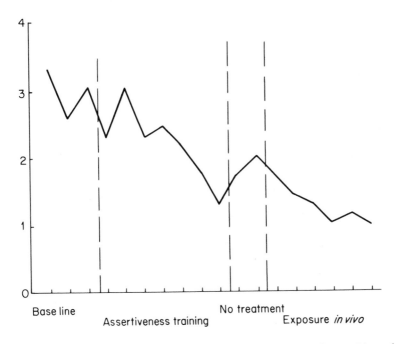

Figure 3.   Weekly means of daily ratings of obsessive–compulsive problems (range
0–8)

Maudsley Obsessional Compulsive Inventory (Hodgson and Rachman, 1977), Self-
rating Depression Scale (Zung, 1965) and a Dutch Assertiveness scale (LAS).
Treatment by assertive training led not only to less anxiety experienced in social
situations   (LAS-tension),   but   the   improvement   generalized   to   the
obsessive–compulsive problems and depression. The second treatment (exposure *in
vivo*) could add little to the improvements already achieved.

The results of this case study are consistent with our earlier findings in showing
that assertive training may lead to a reduction of the obsessive–compulsive problems.
In a recent study by Emmelkamp and Van de Heyden (1980) assertive training was
applied to six patients with harming obsessions. It was hypothesized that patients
with harming obsessions could not handle their aggressive feelings adequately.
Therefore, we expected that assertive training could be a valuable treatment for such
patients. Results of this study indicate that assertive training was at least as effective
as thought stopping. However, it would be inadvisable to treat these results as
demonstrating the usefulness of assertive training for most obsessive–compulsive
patients. The data and arguments presented here only stresses the importance of a
functional analysis.

For the sake of simplicity I have confined this discussion to the relationship
between unassertiveness and obsessive-compulsive problems. However, a functional

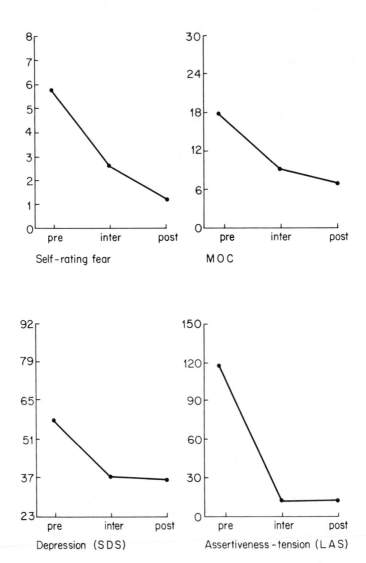

Figure 4. Relative contribution of assertiveness training (pre-test–intermediate test) and exposure *in vivo* (intermediate test–post-test). (Range LAS 0–200)

analysis might reveal other therapeutic strategies as well. In several obsessive–compulsive cases we found that the rituals served the function of avoiding such painful emotions as depression, loneliness, or grief. In passing, it is worth mentioning that in a certain number of our cases the obsessive–compulsive problems develop soon after the death of a relative or an acquaintaince. In such cases prolonged emotional confrontation to painful experiences in the past that are cognitively avoided by the patient might be more useful than treatment that focuses directly on the obsessive–compulsive problems. Although we found this treatment approach to be useful in a few selected cases where previous treatment with exposure had only meagre results, there is little reason to recommend this approach. It has to be said that the use of such painful procedures can be justified only on the grounds of demonstrable therapeutic success.

To summarize, I have attempted to show with a few clinical impressions that we need to look beyond the concept of anxiety reduction as currently used in behavioural theorizing about the functioning of obsessive–compulsive problems. In my opinion, the obsessive–compulsive problems may serve other functions as well. If the alternatives raised here are replicated and confirmed, the theory needs to accommodate these findings. For clinical purposes, it is well to remember that a functional analysis should be a condition *sine qua non* for each case referred for treatment.

REFERENCES

Boersma, K., Den Hengst, G., Dekker, J., and Emmelkamp, P. M. G. (1975) Exposure and response prevention in the natural environment: A comparison with obsessive–compulsive patients. *Behaviour Research and Therapy*, **14**, 19–24.

Cooper, J. (1970) The Leyton Obsessional Inventory. *Psychological Medicine*, **1**, 48–64.

Emmelkamp, P. M. G. (1979) The behavioural study of clinical phobias, in: Hersen, M., Eisler, R. M., and Miller, P. M. (eds.) *Progress in Behavior Modification*. Academic Press, New York, Vol. 8, pp. 55–125.

Emmelkamp, P. M. G. (1981) Anxiety and fear, in Bellack, A., Hersen, M., and Kazdin, A. (eds.), *International Handbook of Behavior Modification and Therapy*. Vol. II. Plenum Press, New York (in press).

Emmelkamp, P. M. G. (1982) Obsessive–compulsive disorders: A clinical research approach, in: Hand, I. (ed.) *Obsessions and Compulsions: Recent Advances in Behavioral Analysis and Therapy*. Springer, New York (in press).

Emmelkamp, P. M. G., and Kraanen, J. (1977) Therapist controlled exposure *in vivo* versus self-controlled exposure *in vivo*: A comparison with obsessive–compulsive patients. *Behaviour Research and Therapy*, **15**, 491–495.

Emmelkamp, P. M. G., Kuipers, A., and Eggeraat, J. (1978) Cognitive modification versus prolonged exposure *in vivo*: A comparison with agoraphobics. *Behaviour Research and Therapy*, **16**, 33–41.

Emmelkamp, P. M. G., and Kwee, K. G. (1977) Obsessional ruminations: A comparison between thought-stopping and prolonged exposure in imagination. *Behaviour Research and Therapy*, **15**, 441–444.

Emmelkamp, P. M. G., Van der Helm, M., Van Zanten, B., and Plochg, I. (1980) Treatment of obsessive–compulsive patients: The contribution of self-instructional training to the effectiveness of exposure. *Behaviour Research and Therapy*, **18**, 61–66.

Emmelkamp, P. M. G., and Van der Heyden, H. (1980) The treatment of harming obsessions. *Behavioral Analysis and Modification*, **4(1)** 28–35.

Hodgson, R. J., and Rachman, S. (1977) Obsessional compulsive complaints. *Behaviour Research and Therapy*, **15,** 389–395.

Meichenbaum, D. H. (1975) Self-instructional methods, in Kanfer, F. H. and Goldstein, A. P. (eds.), *Helping People Change*. Pergamon Press, New York, pp. 357–391.

Watson, J. P., and Marks, I. (1971) Relevant and irrelevant fear in flooding: A cross-over study of phobic patients. *Behavior Therapy*, **2,** 275–295.

Zung, W. W. K. (1965) A self-rating depression scale. *Archives of General Psychiatry*, **12,** 63–70.

Learning Theory Approaches to Psychiatry
Edited by John Boulougouris
© 1982 John Wiley & Sons Ltd

12. DEPRESSION, HABITUATION, AND TREATMENT OUTCOME IN OBSESSIVE–COMPULSIVES

Edna Foa, Jonathan Grayson, and Gail Steketee

The joint occurrence of depression and obsessive–compulsive neurosis has been noted by numerous authors, (Beech, 1971; Cammer, 1973; Kendell and DiScipio, 1970; Lewis, 1936, Mellett, 1974; Rachman, 1976; Walker and Beech, 1969). That Rachman and Hodgson devoted an entire chapter to this subject in their recent book (Rachman and Hodgson, 1980) testifies to the wide recognition of the link between these two psychopathological manifestations. Indeed, most obsessive–compulsives evidence at least some degree of depression (Foa and Goldstein, 1978; Marks *et al.* 1980; Rachman *et al.*, 1979).

While the exact nature of this relationship is still unclear, several authors have noted that the presence of severe depression hinders the effectiveness of treatment by exposure and response prevention (Foa *et al.*, 1979; Marks, 1973, 1977). Likewise, the temporary interference of depressive mood with progress during treatment, resulting at times in loss of previous gains, was described by Rachman and Hodgson (1980, p. 80).

Obversely, the reduction of depression through the administration of clomipramine was found to enhance the effects of behavioural treatment. In a sample of 40 obsessive–compulsives treated by exposure and response prevention with and without clomipramine, clomipramine reduced depression, whereas behavioural treatment affected obsessive–compulsive symptomatology (Rachman *et al.*, 1979). Depressed patients who received clomipramine became less depressed and gained more from exposure treatment than did those who received placebo. This difference became more marked at follow-up, the placebo group evidencing a relapse while the clomipramine group maintained their gains. However, clomipramine did not improve upon placebo in reducing obsessive–compulsive symptoms and depression in the group that evidenced only mild initial depression (Marks *et al.*, 1980). Thus, these results support the contention that depression interferes with treatment gains.

In discussing the failure to respond to behavioural treatment, Foa (1979) suggested that severely depressed obsessive–compulsives exhibited less habituation of subjective anxiety both within and between exposure sessions. She proposed that this failure to habituate was responsible for their non-responsiveness to exposure and response prevention treatment. In the present chapter, we will further examine the relationship between depression, habituation, and treatment outcome.

METHOD

Patients

Forty-seven obsessive–compulsive patients participating in various studies conducted in the Behavior Therapy Unit during the past six years (Foa, 1979; Foa and Chambless, 1978; Foa and Goldstein, 1978; Foa et al., 1980a, b) constitutes the sample of the present study. Patients included in it conformed to the following criteria: (1) Presence of identifiable discomfort producing stimuli followed by distinct ritualistic behaviours or urges to emit them. (2) Obsessive–compulsive symptoms severe enough to cause considerable interference in everyday functioning and constituting the main complaint. (3) Absence of overt psychosis. (4) Agreement to participate in the treatment programme. The present study thus included 22 males and 25 females, ranging in age from 16 years to 58 years with a mean of 33 years. Mean duration of symptoms was 10.3 years with a range of one year to 30 years, 33 patients had washing compulsions and 13 manifested checking rituals.

Treatment

Each patient was first interviewed by a senior psychologist who determined her or his suitability for treatment according to the four criteria described above. All patients received prolonged exposure and supervised response prevention (for more details see Foa and Goldstein, 1978). Of the 47 patients, 23 received ten to 15 daily sessions of both imaginal and *in vivo* exposure to feared items, each session lasting two hours. Nine were treated with ten daily sessions of response prevention and exposure *in vivo* only. Another ten patients were given 20 treatment sessions in a cross-over design: five of them received ten sessions of exposure *in vivo* with no response prevention, followed by ten sessions of exposure *in vivo* and response prevention; the remaining five received two weeks of response prevention only, followed by ten sessions of combined treatment (Foa et al., 1980a). Five additional patients were treated by 15 sessions of response prevention and exposure *in vivo*. During treatment by exposure all patients were asked to practise for four hours per day by exposing themselves to the same items that had been employed in the session.

    Patients who received treatment by *in vivo* exposure (with no presentation of imaginal scenes) reported their level of anxiety, on a 0 to 100 scale, every ten minutes during each session. Those who received exposure in imagination as well as *in vivo* rated their anxiety level during imaginal exposure only. These imaginal data were not included in the analysis of habituation since the present chapter is concerned with the relationship between depression and habituation during *in vivo* exposure.

Measures

Depression Level of depression at pre-treatment was rated on a 0 to 8 Likert-like scale (0—no depression and 8—severe depression) by both the patient and an independent assessor. To enhance the validity and reliability of this measure these ratings were averaged. Using the Spearman Brown prophecy formula, the reliability of this combined score was 0.74.

Outcome measures On the basis of a 45–60 minute interview the independent assessor rated each patient on severity of compulsions and obsessions. Both scales ranged from 0 to 8, 0 representing no symptoms and 8 representing severe symptomatology. The assessor was instructed to collect information on the patients' behaviour, lifestyle, performance in her/his different roles, etc. These data provided the basis for his ratings. (He was specifically instructed to avoid requests of self-rating from the patients.) Assessments were conducted at pre-treatment, post-treatment and at three, six, twelve, 24, and 36 months. The data reported in the present chapter include the most recent follow-up; the mean was 12.5 months with a range of three to 36 months. Follow-up data were not available for some patients.

Habituation

To assess habituation, subjective anxiety during two sessions of exposure *in vivo* were examined: the session in which patients were first exposed to their most feared item or situation, and the tenth treatment session. The average number of sessions between these two points in treatment was 6.4.

Habituation within sessions This was defined as the percentage change between the highest anxiety level reported during the first *in vivo* presentation of the most feared item and the lowest level following it during this same session.

Habituation between sessions This was defined as the percentage change between the initial highest anxiety level and the highest anxiety level reported during the tenth session of *in vivo* exposure.

A word of caution The measures of depression, habituation, and outcome reported in this chapter are less rigorous than desirable. The manner in which exposure was conducted was tailored to clinical rather than research requirements. Thus, the length of exposure to any particular item was not kept constant across sessions or subjects; rather, when patients habituated to a given situation a new one was introduced within the same session. With respect to outcome measures, these were based upon assessor's evaluation only; the addition of self-report and behavioural measures would have been preferable. Although in our on-going studies such data are being collected, the only measures common to all 47 subjects included in the present study were the assessor's ratings. As to our measure of depression, the reliability of the combined rating was only 0.74. Inclusion of other measures of depression would have been desirable to increase the reliability.

RESULTS

On the basis of their initial depression score patients were divided into three groups in the following manner. The mean score and standard deviation for all patients were computed, yielding a mean of 4.12 and S.D. of 2.10. The ten patients who were 1 S.D. above the mean (6.5 and above) comprised the highly-depressed group. The low-depressed group consisted of the ten patients whose score was 1 S.D. below the mean (0–2). The remaining 27 patients constituted the moderately-depressed group (2.5–6).

These three groups did not differ significantly with respect to initial severity of obsessions and compulsions. The mean severity of obsessions was 5.57 for the low-depressed group, 6.93 for the moderately-depressed, and 7.00 for the highly-depressed. The mean severity of compulsions for the three groups was 6.30, 6.90, and 6.77 respectively.

Patients varied with respect to the number of exposure sessions they received (range: 10–20). However, no significant differences were found in the mean number of sessions received by the members of each group. The mean number of sessions for the entire sample was 12.5.

Depression and outcome

To obtain a measure of the magnitude of improvement, the change scores from pre- to post-treatment and from pre-treatment to follow-up were divided by the pre-treatment score and thus converted into percentage improvement scores. This was done separately for obsessions and compulsions, resulting in four scores for each patient. (For those patients who did not have follow-up evaluation, only two scores were obtained.) Higher positive scores indicate greater improvement.

The mean percentage change on obsessions and compulsions at post-treatment and at follow-up was calculated separately for the three groups. These means are shown in Figures 1 and 2.

To test the hypothesis that depressed patients improve less than the non-depressed ones t-tests were computed for all possible comparisons. These are given in Table 1. Inspection of this Table supports our hypothesis. The highly-depressed patients improved less than did the low-depressed ones on both obsessions and compulsions at post-treatment and at follow-up. They also showed less improvement than the moderately-depressed patients at follow-up on both obsessions and compulsions, evidencing a loss of treatment gains. Indeed, only in the highly-depressed group there

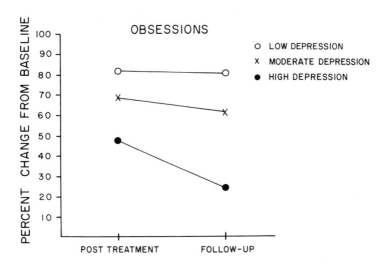

Figure 1.   Mean percentage improvement for low, moderate, and highly depressed patients on assessors' ratings of obsessions at post-treatment and at follow-up

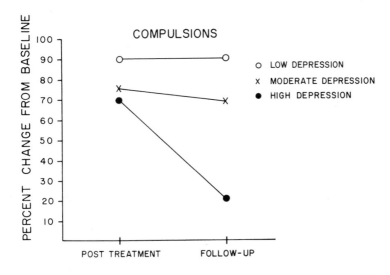

Figure 2.   Mean percentage improvement for low, moderate, and highly depressed patients on assessors' ratings of compulsions at post-treatment and at follow-up

Table 1.　Planned comparisons* between levels of depression for percentage change of obsessions and compulsions

Dependent Variables	Percentage Change	Low vs. Moderate	Depression Moderate vs. high	Low vs. high
Obsessions	post-treatment	$t = 1.37$ df 35	$t = 1.65$ df 35	$t = 3.05‡$ df 18
	follow-up	$t = 1.37$ df 31	$t = 2.38†$ df 29	$t = 4.24‡$ df 16
Compulsions	post-treatment	$t = 1.50$ df 35	$t = 0.62$ df 35	$t = 2.47†$ df 18
	follow-up	$t = 18$ df 28	$t = 1.78†$ df 27	$t = 2.44†$ df 15

*All p values are one tailed-test
†$p < 0.05$
‡$p < 0.01$

Table 2.　Correlations between treatment outcome and depression, habituation, initial severity of symptoms, and initial level of anxiety

	Obsessions Percentage change		Compulsions Percentage change	
	Post-treatment	Follow-up	Post-treatment	Follow-up
Depression	-0.36 $n = 47$ $p = 0.006$	-0.41 $n = 39$ $p = 0.005$	-0.24 $n = 7$ $p = 0.05$	-0.30 $n = 38$ $p = 0.03$
Habituation within sessions	NS	NS	NS	NS
Habituation between sessions	0.43 $n = 22$ $p = 0.025$	0.43 $n = 19$ $p = 0.02$	0.36 $n = 22$ $p = 0.05$	NS
Initial severity of obsessions	NS	NS	NS	NS
Initial severity of compulsions	NS	NS	NS	NS
Initial level of anxiety to most feared item	NS	NS	NS	NS

was a significant increase in obsessions from post-treatment to follow-up ($t = 3.61$, df 7, $p < 0.01$). With regard to compulsions, the same trend was observed, although this difference failed to reach significance ($t = 1.92$, df 7, $p < 0.1$). (See Figures 1 and 2). The moderately-depressed patients did not differ from the mildly-depressed ones at any point.

To further explore the relationship between depression and treatment outcome, correlation coefficients between depression and each of the four outcome scores were computed. These are presented in Table 2. As predicted depression was significantly and negatively correlated with percentage change on obsessions and compulsions, both at post-treatment and at follow-up. In summary, highly-depressed patients gained less from treatment than low-depressed patients. Moreover, they relapsed more than did either the low- or moderately-depressed ones.

Depression and habituation

Complete data for habituation were available for only 22 of the 23 patients who received exposure *in vivo* without imaginal exposure. Five of these were in the low depressed group, eleven in the moderately depressed, and six in the highly depressed group. The point in treatment at which patients were exposed to their most feared item varied across patients; consequently, the number of sessions that elapsed between the two sessions used to compute the rate of inter-session habituation also varied across patients. The mean for these sessions was therefore computed separately for each group. Differences between groups would have raised the possibility that differences in habituation could be attributed to the varied length of exposure time. Utilizing *t*-tests, no significant differences among groups were found.

To test the hypothesis that depressed patients habituate less than non-depressed, the mean percentage change scores of habituation within a session and between sessions were computed separately for each of the three groups. These means are presented in Figure 3.

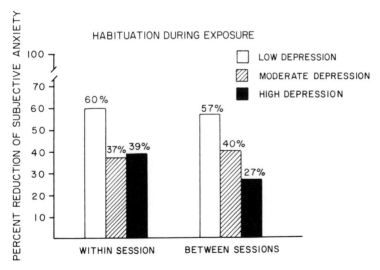

Figure 3.   Mean percentage of habituation of subjective anxiety within and between sessions, for low-, moderate-, and highly-depressed patients

Inspection of this Figure reveals that the least depressed group habituated more within a session than did the most depressed group (mean percentage changes of 60 and 39 respectively). The degree of habituation observed in the moderately-depressed group (37%) was unexpectedly similar to that of the highly-depressed. Although the differences between the high- and low-depressed groups were in the predicted direction, they failed to reach significance on t-tests. Similarly, no significant differences between the moderate and the high groups were found. Only the difference between the means of the low- and moderate-depressed patients was significant ($t = 2.77$, df 14, $p<0.01$).

With respect to habituation between sessions, the low-depressed group habituated twice as much as the high-depressed group (means of 57% and 27% respectively). The moderately-depressed fell in between with a mean percentage habituation of 40. Thus, the differences between the means were in the predicted direction, although the results of the t-tests were again not significant. It should be noted, however, that the numbers in the high and low group were very small (six and five respectively).

In order to further examine the relationship between depression and habituation within and between sessions correlation coefficients were computed. These are reported in Table 3. Depression was negatively correlated with both habituation within and between sessions, yielding coefficients of -0.33 ($n = 22$, $p = 0.07$) and -0.35 ($n = 22$, $p = 0.06$) respectively. The hypothesis that deficiency in habituation is responsible for the poorer outcome of severely depressed patients received only marginal support.

Table 3. Correlations between depression, initial level of anxiety and habituation

	Habituation within	Habituation between	Depression
Depression	-0.33	-0.35	
	$n = 22$	$n = 22$	—
	$p = 0.07$	$p = 0.06$	
Initial level	-0.33	-0.54	0.61
of anxiety to	$n = 22$	$n = 22$	$n = 22$
most feared item	$p = 0.07$	$p = 0.001$	$p = 0.002$

Habituation and outcome

Our original chain of reasoning was as follows: (1) Depression interferes with habituation; (2) habituation leads to improvement and therefore; (3) depressed patients evidence less improvement. To complete the examination of this proposition the relationship between habituation and outcome remains to be analysed. To this end correlation coefficients were computed between each of the four outcome measures and the two types of habituation. They are reported in Table 2. Intra-session habituation was not related to treatment outcome. However, habituation between sessions did correlate significantly with percentage change in obsessions, both at post-treatment and at follow-up and with percentage change of compulsions at post-treatment. Its correlation with compulsions at follow-up did not reach significance.

Depression, habituation, and initial anxiety to feared stimuli

Habituation and depression were both found to be related to outcome, while the relationship between them was only marginally significant. Therefore the inferior outcome found in depressed patients cannot be attributed solely to their failure to habituate. Nor can the relationship between inter-session habituation and outcome be accounted for by depression alone. What other variables might account for the relationship of depression to outcome?

Since depression was significantly correlated with initial severity of obsessions $(0.29, n = 47, p < 0.025)$, we tested the hypothesis that the inferior outcome of the highly-depressed patients was due to greater initial severity of obsessions. The results did not support this hypothesis. The correlation coefficients of initial severity of obsessions with percentage change on obsessions and compulsions (both at post-test and follow-up) were not significant.

Another measure of severity is the level of initial anxiety reported at the first presentation of the most feared item. We explored the possibility that this measure of severity is related to depression and in turn to habituation and outcome. Specifically, we hypothesized that since depressed patients are thought to have a greater level of sensitivity, depression will be positively correlated with reported initial anxiety. Indeed, the correlation coefficient between these two variables was rather high (0.61) (see Table 3). However, initial anxiety was not significantly correlated with any of the four measures of outcome and therefore cannot directly account for the inferior outcome of depressed patients. On the other hand, initial level of anxiety to the most feared item was significantly and negatively correlated with habituation between sessions (-0.54) but only marginally with habituation within sessions (-0.33) (see Table 3).

The relatively high negative correlation found between inter-session habituation and initial level of anxiety might possibly be an artifact, since one of the two scores used to derive the habituation measure was the initial anxiety score. However, the same score was also used to compute the measure of intra-session habituation, yet the correlation between these two measures was much lower. Therefore, it seems unlikely that the relationship between inter-session habituation and anxiety is artifactual.

Figure 4 illustrates the network of these relationships. It shows that the two best predictors of outcome were level of depression and the degree of habituation between sessions. Habituation, in turn, was related to both initial reported anxiety to most feared stimuli and to depression. When the correlation between initial anxiety and depression was partialled out, no relationship between depression and habituation remained (partial r $= -0.03$). On the other hand, partialling out the relationship

RELATIONSHIP BETWEEN OUTCOME AND DEPRESSION,
HABITUATION, AND INITIAL ANXIETY TO MOST FEARED ITEM

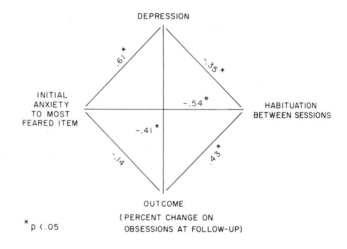

Figure 4. The relationships between percentage improvement on obsessions and depression, inter-session habituation, and initial level of subjective anxiety to most feared situation

between depression and habituation did not significantly affect the correlation between initial level of anxiety and habituation (partial r = − 0.44). In summary, the relationship between depression and inter-session habituation seems due to the fact that both are related to initial anxiety.

As to the relative contribution of depression and habituation in predicting outcome, when the effect of depression is partialled out, the correlation between habituation and outcome is only slightly reduced to 0.33. Likewise, when the effect of habituation is partialled out, the correlation between depression and outcome does not change much (partial r = − 0.30). It follows that habituation and depression seem to affect outcome independently.

DISCUSSION

We hypothesized that severely depressed obsessive–compulsives would not benefit from treatment by exposure and response prevention as much as non-depressed patients. The results confirmed this hypothesis. The highly depressed group showed less percentage change on measures of obsessions and compulsions than did the low depressed group. Moreover, of the three groups only the highly depressed evidenced a relapse at follow-up: 22% of the low depressed and 33% of the moderately depressed group failed to benefit from treatment or relapsed at follow-up. In contrast, this figure was 62% for the highly depressed group.

These results are congruent with clinical observations reported by Marks (1973), Foa and Goldstein (1978), Foa (1979), and Rachman and Hodgson (1980). They are also congruent with Boulougouris' (1977) finding of a high negative correlation between depression and the interference score of the Leyton Obsessional Inventory at follow-up. However, he reported no relationship between depression and clinical ratings of main obsession. Our highly-depressed group seems to be similar to the subsample of depressed obsessive–compulsives reported by Marks *et al.* (1980). It is, therefore, of interest to note that the five patients of their group who did not receive clomipramine showed a pattern similar to that found in our highly-depressed patients. Both evidenced inferior outcome at post-treatment and a relapse at follow-up.

A negative relationship between depression and outcome was also reported by Zitrin *et al.* (1980) for agoraphobics, on global improvement ratings by therapist and assessor as well as on patient self-ratings. Thus, the interference of depression with treatment efficacy may occur across diagnostic categories.

The hypothesis that habituation is related to treatment outcome was supported only for inter-session habituation. When improvement on obsessions is conceptualized as a long-term habituation of fear, it stands to reason that the degree of inter-session habituation, as defined here (across a mean of 6.4 sessions), should constitute a better predictor of outcome than the degree of habituation within two hours time. These results thus support Foa's (1979) contention that intra-session habituation is not a sufficient condition for symptom reduction.

With respect to the hypothesis that depression interferes with habituation, a trend in the predicted direction was evident but was only marginally significant. Since the magnitude of the relationship found between depression and habituation was not sufficient to account for the poorer outcome observed in depressed obsessive–compulsives, we explored other potential intervening variables. These further analyses were performed in order to generate hypotheses for future research rather than to arrive at definitive conclusions.

It was then found that the relationship between depression and habituation is mediated by the high initial level of anxiety associated with depression. Indeed, Lader and Wing (1969) reported that agitated, depressed patients showed greater arousal and less habituation to neutral stimuli on GSR measures than did normals. Further support for the contention that initial high level of anxiety hinders habituation comes from a recent study by Grey *et al.* (1979) with phobic subjects. These authors found that subjects who were exposed to situations which aroused moderate anxiety evidenced greater habituation on subjective ratings of anxiety than did those exposed to highly disturbing situations. As in our study they found this difference for inter-session but not for intra-session habituation. Interestingly, in both studies the initial level of anxiety during exposure was not related to outcome. More generally, high intensity stimuli appear to hinder habituation in animals (Davis and

Wagner, 1969; Groves and Thompson, 1970) as well as in humans (O'Gorman and Jamieson, 1975; Grayson, 1979). Thus, the inverse relationship between initial responsiveness and habituation may well be of wider validity, involving both cognitive and physiological responses.

Since the effect of depression on treatment outcome is mediated by habituation to only a small extent, what other variables may affect this relationship? One such variable may be decreased compliance with treatment demands in depressed obsessive–compulsives. Indeed Marks *et al.* (1980) found that clomipramine (which reduced depressed mood) increased compliance both during and between sessions. We did not observe our depressed patients to be less compliant during treatment, but their high rate of relapse might have reflected non-comliance with post-treatment instructions.

It is also possible that depressed obsessive–compulsives perceive themselves as more helpless (Seligman, 1975), and/or less efficacious (Bandura, 1977) than non-depressed ones, resulting in lower expectations of improvement and thus interfering with treatment gains. Additionally, depressed patients have been found to attribute success to external sources and failure to internal sources (Raps *et al.*, 1980; Seligman *et al.*, 1979). External attribution of therapeutic gains (to drugs) has been shown to result in relapse (Davison and Valins, 1969). Perhaps, then, the highly-depressed obsessive–compulsives attribute their limited gains to external sources (e.g. therapist control, treatment regimen) and therefore evidence less improvement and more relapses than non-depressed patients.

It is quite clear from the preceding discussion that more than one variable accounts for the inverse relationship between depression and treatment outcome in obsessive–compulsives. Identification of such variables will enable us to modify our present procedures in order to maximize treatment efficacy. For example, if the finding that initial level of reported anxiety interferes with habituation is substantiated, exposure should be more gradual when patients evidence high initial level of subjective anxiety, using the desensitization model (Wolpe, 1958, 1973). Likewise, if cognitive variables such as expectancy and attribution are found to vary with depression, it will be expedient to incorporate procedures which affect such variables into treatment programmes for these patients.

In summary, habituation does not seem to be the kingpin of the relationship between depression and treatment outcome in obsessive–compulsives. Hopefully, our preliminary results and the hypothesis we derived will stimulate further research of this problem.

NOTES

Preparation of this paper was supported by NIMH Grant No. MH 31634-02 awarded to the first author. The authors wish to express their appreciation to Abby Rosenfield for her helpful remarks.
    Requests for reprints should be addressed to Edna B. Foa, Ph.D., Temple University, Department of Psychiatry, c/o E.P.P.I., 3300 Henry Ave., Philadelphia, Pa., 19129 USA.

REFERENCES

Bandura, A. (1977) Self efficacy: Toward a unifying theory of behavioral change. *Psychological Review*, **84**, 191–215.

Beech, H. R. (1971) Ritualistic activity in obsessional patients. *Journal of Psychosomatic Research*, **15**, 417–422.

Boulougouris, J. (1977) Variables affecting the behavior modification of obsessive–compulsive patients treated by flooding, in Boulougouris, J. C., and Rabavilas, A. D. (eds.) *Treatment of Phobic and Obsessive–Compulsive Disorders*. Pergamon Press, New York, pp. 73–84.

Cammer, L. (1973) Antidepressants as a prophylaxis against depression in the obsessive–compulsive person. *Psychosomatics*, **14**, 201–206.

Davis, M., and Wagner, A. R. (1966) Habituation of the startle response under incremental sequence of stimulus intensities. *Journal of Comparative and Physiological Psychology*, **67**, 486–492.

Davison, G. C., and Valins, R. (1969) Maintenance of self-attributed and drug attributed behavior change. *Journal of Personality and Social Psychology*, **11**, 25–33.

Foa, E. B. (1979) Failure in treating obsessive–compulsives. *Behaviour Research and Therapy*, **17**, 169–176.

Foa, E. B., and Chambless, D. L. (1978) Habituation of subjective anxiety during flooding in imagery. *Behaviour Research and Therapy*, **16**, 391–399.

Foa, E. B., and Goldstein, A. (1978) Continuous exposure and complete response prevention in the treatment of obsessive–compulsive neurosis. *Behavior Therapy*, **9**, 821–829.

Foa, E. B., Steketee, G., and Groves, G. A. (1979) Use of behavioral therapy and imipramine: A case of obsessive–compulsive neurosis with severe depression. *Behavior Modification*, **3**, 419–430.

Foa, E. B., Steketee, G., and Milby, J. B. (1980a) Differential effects of exposure and response prevention in obsessive–compulsive washers. *Journal of Consulting and Clinical Psychology*, **48**, 71–79.

Foa, E. B., Steketee, G., Turner, R. M., and Fischer, S. C. (1980b) Effects of imaginal exposure to feared disasters. *Behaviour Research and Therapy*, **18**, 449–455.

Grayson, J. B. (1979) *Orienting and defensive responses in phobic imagery and the incremental stimulus intensity effect*. Paper presented at the Thirteenth Annual Meeting of the Association for the Advancement of Behavior Therapy. San Francisco.

Grey, S., Sartory, G., and Rachman, S. (1979) Synchronous and desynchronous changes during fear reduction. *Behaviour Research and Therapy*, **17**, 137–147.

Groves, P. M., and Thompson, R. F. (1970) Habituation: A dual process theory. *Psychological Review*, **77**, 419–450.

Kendell, R. E., and DiScipio, W. J. (1970) Obsessional symptoms and obsessional personality traits in patients with depressive illness. *Psychological Medicine*, **1**, 65–72.

Lader, M. H., and Wing, L. (1969) Physiological measures in agitated and retarded depressed patients. *Journal of Psychiatric Research*, **7**, 89–100.

Lewis, A. J. (1936) Problems of obsessional illness. *Proceedings of the Royal Society of Medicine*, **24**, 325–336.

Marks, I. (1973) New approaches to the treatment of obsessive–compulsive disorders. *The Journal of Nervous and Mental Disease*, **156**, 420–426.

Marks, I. (1977) Recent results of behavioural treatments of phobias and obsessions. *Journal of Internal Medicine Research*, **5**, 16–21.

Marks, I., Stern, R. S., Mawson, D., Cobb, J., and McDonald, R. (1980) Clomipramine and exposure for obsessive–compulsive rituals: I. *British Journal of Psychiatry*, **136**, 1–25.

Mellet, P. G. (1974) The clinical problem, in Beech, H. R. (ed.) *Obsessional states*. Methuen, London, pp. 55–94.

O'Gorman, J. G., and Jamieson, R. D. (1975) The incremental stimulus intensity effect and habituation of autonomic responses in man. *Physiological Psychology*, **3**, 385–389.

Rachman, S. (1976) Obsessional–compulsive checking. *Behaviour Research and Therapy*, **14**, 269–277.

Rachman, S., Cobb, J., Grey, S., McDonald, B., Mawson, D., Sartory, G., and Stern, R. (1979) The behavioural treatment of obsessional–compulsive disorders, with and without clomipramine. *Behaviour Research and Therapy*, **17**, 467–478.

Rachman, S., and Hodgson, R. J. (1980) *Obsessions and compulsions*. Prentice Hall, Englewood Cliffs, New Jersey.

Raps, C., Abramson, L. Y., and Seligman, M. E. P. (1980) *Depressive attributional style in affective disorders*. Unpublished manuscript University of Pennsylvania.

Seligman, M. E. P. (1975) *Helplessness*. Freeman, San Francisco.

Seligman, M. E. P., Abramson, L. Y., Semmel, A., and Von-Bayer, C. (1979) Depressive attributional style. *Journal of Abnormal Psychology*, **88**, 242–247.

Walker, V. J., and Beech, H. R. (1969) Mood state and the ritualistic behaviour of obsessional patients. *Journal of Psychiatry*, **115**, 1261–1263.

Wolpe, J. (1958) *Psychotherapy by reciprocal inhibition*. Stanford University Press, Stanford.

Wolpe, J. (1973) *The practice of behaviour therapy*. Pergamon Press, London.

Zitrin, C. M., Klein, D. F., and Woerner, M. G. (1980) Treatment of agoraphobia with group exposure *in vivo* and imipramine. *Archives of General Psychiatry*, **37**, 63–72.

Learning Theory Approaches to Psychiatry
Edited by John Boulougouris
© 1982 John Wiley & Sons Ltd

13. EXPERIENCED VERSUS INEXPERIENCED THERAPISTS IN THE TREATMENT WITH EXPOSURE *IN VIVO*

John Boulougouris, Andreas Rabavilas, John Liappas, and Dimitri Tabouratzis

Although there are marked differences regarding the definition of psychotherapy, most reports agree that the patient–therapist relationship is an important contributor to psychotherapeutic outcome (Truax, 1961; Goldstein *et al.*, 1966). In this context, variables concerning the patient, the therapist, the technique employed, and the patient–therapist similarity have been investigated, but so far, the critical dimensions of the relationship itself remain speculative (Gardner, 1964). While this state of affairs applies to most of the traditional psychotherapies, the psychotherapeutic relationship in a behaviour therapy setting has been given little attention since the early report of Wilson and Hannon (1968). However, there appears, quite frequently, in the literature some indirect information suggesting that certain patient–therapist variables may operate during behavioural psychotherapy. In particular such variables are: the quality of personal contact, therapist's verbal cues, and his actions, which may trigger off and facilitate the practice of counteravoidance behaviour. This appears to apply particularly to exposure treatments. The therapist with exposure *in vivo* techniques, for example, has to intervene promptly and sometimes vigorously in order to deal with emerging behaviours which are occasionally undesirable or beyond the therapeutic targets. Such intervention, which reflects the therapist's own style of working, may take many forms: from deciding how to deal with a patient's sudden resistance to face an avoidance situation to increasing a patient's motivation or minimizing his dependence on the therapist (Mathews, 1977). Thus, the therapist has to become a source of both discriminative and reinforcing stimuli (Staats, 1964), the over-all identity of which could be reduced to a common denominator, which in fact is his relationship with the patient (Foa and Steketee, 1979).

From our personal experience in the field and others' findings as well (R. Hodgson, personal communication, 1976; Mathews *et al.*, 1976), it has been suggested that the style of the therapist or therapist identity might account for the outcome with exposure treatments on neurotic patients. Such properties, however, are considered by others as less important when structured behaviour techniques are employed (Emmelkamp and Kraanen, 1977).

Having made the assumption that the relationship is of some importance in this type of treatment a retrospective evaluation of some therapist qualities in relation to therapeutic change was carried out in 36 phobic and obsessive–compulsive patients treated with flooding type exposure *in vivo* (Rabavilas *et al.*, 1979). In that study some indications for good outcome derived from patient's judgement regarding the therapist's general attitude towards them were: therapist's respect, understanding, and interest towards them. On the contrary, gratification of patient's dependency needs, permissiveness, tolerance, and neutral attitude towards them appeared to carry an adverse effect.

Since this type of retrospective assessment was crude, it was decided to investigate in a prospective study the patient–therapist relationship by comparing the effects of experienced and inexperienced therapists on neurotic patients undertaking *in vivo* exposure therapy. The present chapter deals with some of the findings derived from this study.

Ten patients were treated by means of a factorial 2×2 design. Five of these patients suffered from agoraphobia and five from obsessive–compulsive disorder. All patients had to agree to the conditions of the trial i.e. the change of therapists. Patients' mean age was 33.5 years (S.D. = 7.8) and mean duration of their illness was 7.3 years (S.D. = 6.1).

After the pre-treatment screening patients were allocated in a random order to experienced or inexperienced therapists. After three or four preparatory interviews and an interval of one week the first therapist administered three treatment sessions three times a week (Table 1). After an interval of one week, the treatment was carried out by a second therapist who again in one week's time gave three treatment sessions. That is, each patient had in all three preparatory interviews and six treatment sessions, three from one therapist and three from the other. The three preparatory sessions were given by the first order therapist depending upon the allocation. The second therapist was introduced by the first therapist who also informed him about the patient's problem and the symptoms treated by him. The treatment procedure was carried out on similar lines by both therapists and was that of exposure *in vivo* with flooding plus modelling. Each session lasted for 60 minutes. It is obvious that the *in vivo* session had to vary for each patient. In order to keep the treatment procedure similar for both therapists each therapist prepared for his successor a handbook defining precisely what he had done and what was left to be done. All inexperienced therapists were supervised by the senior author.

Assessment was made by the patient and independent assessor one week after the third preparatory session (baseline assessment) and after the third and sixth treatment session using five-point rating scales regarding: (1) the main complaint (phobia or obsession); (2) the total complaint, i.e. the main symptom plus four other symptoms; (3) anxiety; and (4) depression. Patients completed on a five-point scale their

Table 1. Flow diagram of the study

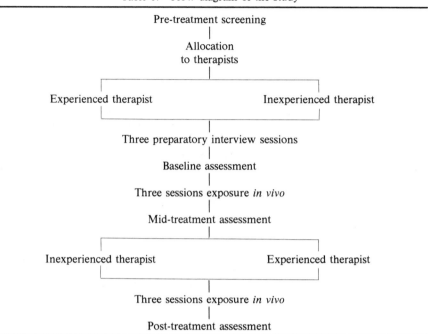

Pre-treatment screening

Allocation
to therapists

Experienced therapist   Inexperienced therapist

Three preparatory interview sessions

Baseline assessment

Three sessions exposure *in vivo*

Mid-treatment assessment

Inexperienced therapist   Experienced therapist

Three sessions exposure *in vivo*

Post-treatment assessment

satisfaction from each therapist at the end of the therapy (0 indicating the highest satisfaction and 4 dissatisfaction). Within treatment sessions assessments were also made, during the third baseline session and during the third and sixth treatment session. The independent assessor was present during these sessions and both he and the patient completed semantic differential scales in order to assess evaluative changes regarding attitudes towards therapist. The assessor rated in addition evaluative scales regarding the 'over-all relationship', 'warmth', 'dependence', and 'identification'. The independent assessor was also asked to make reports on various patient–therapist responses indicating psychological support and the ways such support was provided. Patients were asked for written reports on their therapists and they had to decide with whom they would like to continue therapy after the end of the trial. Patients and therapists also completed before treatment the Eysenck Personality Inventory (Eysenck and Eysenck, 1964) and the State-Trait Anxiety Inventory (Spielberger *et al.*, 1970). The therapist completed as well eight-point rating scales for patient's motivation and how much his/her family interferes with the problem (0 indicating the highest motivation or lack of family interference).

The experienced therapists were qualified psychiatrists with previous experience in behaviour therapy techniques of at least one year. The inexperienced therapists were trainees in psychiatry or psychologists and did not have any previous experience in any type of psychotherapy but had shown interest in behaviour therapy and asked to treat a suitable case.

Analysis of variance was performed by inserting the change scores for improvement between pre- and post-third-treatment session versus post-third and post-sixth- treatment session. The effects of experienced versus inexperienced therapists were also computed as well as the type of the patients (phobics versus obsessives).

The effects of experienced compared to inexperienced therapists on behavioural measures according to both the patients' and the assessors' ratings before and after treatment are illustrated on Figure 1. Although an over-all significant reduction after treatment compared to pre-treatment scores was found on main and total complaint, no differences between experienced and inexperienced therapists were detected. Insignificant changes were also found on anxiety and depression ratings by patients and assessors. The results of the ANOVA in main complaint are presented on Table 2. A significant first order effect ($p < 0.001$) is revealed on both patients' and assessors' ratings. Similar findings are revealed with respect to total complaint (Table 3).

Less satisfaction according to patients' ratings were obtained from inexperienced ($m = 2.5$) than from experienced therapists ($m = 1.4$). Inexperienced therapists rated

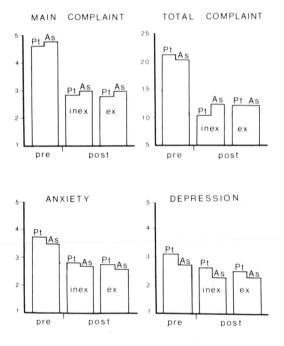

Figure 1.   The effects of experienced and inexperienced therapists on behavioural measures after treatment. Patients' (Pt) and assessors' (As) ratings

Table 2. Analysis of variance on change scores in main complaint

| Experienced first order | | Inexperienced first order | | Source of variance | ANOVA | | | |
Pre–Post 3rd	3rd–Post 6th	Pre–Post 3rd	3rd–Post 6th		SS	DF	MS	F
Patient's ratings								
2	−1	2	1	A	18.05	1	18.05	34.381*
2	0	1	0	B	0.45	1	0.45	0.857
2	0	3	0	AB	0.05	1	0.05	0.095
1	0	3	−1	Within cell	8.4	16	0.225	
2	0	1	1					
Assessor's ratings								
2	0	2	0	A	12.8	1	12.8	17.655*
2	0	3	−1	B	0.8	1	0.8	1.103
0	1	3	0	AB	0.8	1	0.8	1.103
1	−1	2	1	Within cell	11.6	16	0.725	
2	1	1	1					

Factors
A = Pre–Post 3rd vs. 3rd–Post 6th
B = Exp. vs. Inexp.
* $p < 0.001$

Table 3. Analysis of variance on change scores in total complaint

| | Experienced first order | | Inexperienced first order | | Source of variance | ANOVA | | | |
	Pre–Post 3rd	3rd–Post 6th	Pre–Post 3rd	3rd–Post 6th		SS	DF	MS	F
Patient's ratings									
	12	−4	13	3	A	441.8	1	441.8	40.377*
	10	0	3	0	B	3.2	1	3.2	0.292
	11	1	12	−4	AB	0.8	1	0.8	0.073
	5	0	14	0	Within cell	175.2	16	10.95	
	5	1	7	1					
Assessor's ratings									
	12	1	8	8	A	130.05	1	130.05	9.493*
	10	0	9	−3	B	1.25	1	1.25	0.091
	2	2	5	0	AB	2.45	1	2.45	0.179
	2	2	3	7	Within cell	219.2	16	13.7	
	10	2	10	1					

Factors

A = Pre–Post 3rd vs. 3rd–6th changes

B = Exp. vs. Inexp.

* $p < 0.001$

their patients as being less motivated for treatment (m = 1.9) than experienced therapists did (m = 1.5). Family interference in patients' psychopathology was rated as greater by inexperienced (m = 3.7) than experienced therapists (m = 2.8). All the above differences were not significant.

Therapists' EPI and STAI scores were found to be within the limits suggested for an average population. Patients' high scores in neuroticism (m = 18), state-anxiety (m = 59.1), and trait-anxiety (m = 58.5) were similar to those found in other neurotic patients.

The semantic differentials within treatment sessions did not reveal significant levels. However, a linear regression analysis between improvement scores on main complaint (patients' ratings) and patients' attitudes towards therapists revealed significant negative correlation regarding therapist's 'steadiness' and positive ones regarding him being 'calming' and 'relaxed' (Table 4). Similar analysis regarding the assessor's attitude towards therapist (Table 5) reveals significant negative relations with respect to therapist being 'steady', 'sympathetic', 'fast', and 'good'.

Table 4. Linear regression analysis between improvement scores on main complaint (patients' ratings) and patients' attitudes towards therapists

| | | | | | | Patient no. | | | | | | |
		C1	C2	C3	C4	C5	C6	C7	C8	C9	C10	r
Steady	Imp	2	2	2	1	2	1	3	2	3	1	− 0.53
	Att	7	7	7	7	7	7	7	7	6	7	
Calming	Imp	2	2	2	1	2	1	3	2	3	1	0.56
	Att	7	7	7	4	7	7	7	7	7	6	
Relaxed	Imp	2	2	2	1	2	2	1	3	3	1	0.39
	Att	6	7	7	6	7	6	3	6	6	6	

Table 5. Linear regression analysis between improvement scores on main complaint (assessors' ratings) and assessors' attitudes towards therapist

| | | | | | | Patients no. | | | | | | |
		C1	C2	C3	C4	C5	C6	C7	C8	C9	C10	r
Steady	Imp	2	2	2	3	0	1	3	2	2	1	− 0.42
	Att	6	7	7	6	7	7	5	6	6	7	
Sympathetic	Imp	2	2	2	3	0	1	3	2	2	1	− 0.62
	Att	6	7	7	4	6	7	4	6	6	7	
Fast	Imp	2	2	2	3	0	1	3	2	2	1	− 0.64
	Att	3	6	7	4	7	7	5	6	6	7	
Good	Imp	2	2	2	3	0	1	3	2	2	1	− 0.42
	Att	6	7	7	4	6	6	5	6	6	6	

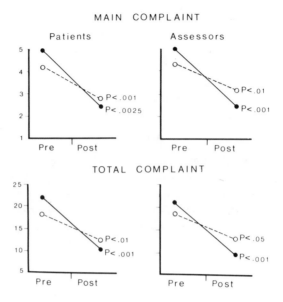

Figure 2.   Mean scores in main and total complaints before and after trial in patients with more (●——●) and less (O - - - - O) positive attitude towards therapist

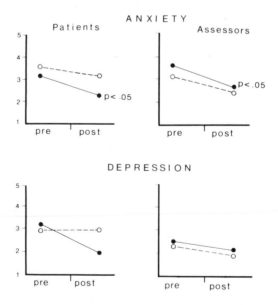

Figure 3.   Mean scores in anxiety and depression before and after trial in patients with more (●——●) and less (O - - - - O) positive attitude towards therapist

In order to obtain a *grosso modo* estimation of the effect of the therapeutic relationship on treatment outcome, the mean evaluation of patients in the 'over-all relationship' as rated by the independent assessors was measured. Patients were allocated to two groups, irrespective to the type of therapist involved: (1) those who scored above mean ('more positive' attitude group, $n = 5$) and (2) those who scored below this mean ('less positive' attitude group, $n = 5$). Patients with a 'less positive' attitude are significantly ($p < 0.057$) more neurotic according to neuroticism EPI scores.

The response to treatment of the 'more' and 'less positive' groups are presented on Figures 2 and 3. Both groups improved significantly on the behavioural measures employed. Comparisons of these two groups regarding their pre- and post-treatment ratings failed to reveal significant differences. However, there is some evidence that patients with a 'more positive' attitude towards their therapists show greater therapeutic change after treatment.

After treatment, most of the patients reported that both therapists were almost equally effective and in fact they could not differentiate the experienced from the inexperienced therapist. They considered that the therapeutic effect was due to the specific technique employed and not to any particular relationship established with the therapist. However, when asked to choose a therapist to continue the treatment with, most of them made their choice without hesitation. In addition, most patients reported excessive dreaming and even daytime fantasies regarding some of their therapists during treatment.

From the results so far in this experiment, it seems likely that the therapeutic interpersonal relationship may be of some importance with this type of behavioural procedure employed, although it is rather early to evaluate these results. A greater number of observations and more follow-up data are needed before one formulates conclusions. But even so, it appears that a number of factors may confound research of this type. The authors feel that the following points should be dealt with in a future investigation:

1. Clarification of concepts: The patient–therapist relationship may be characterized in many ways. Its evaluation regarding therapeutic outcome is not very meaningful if made in ill-defined terms. Thus, clarification of which sorts of relationship are desirable during behaviour therapy and which not, is necessary. If we decided that 'empathy', 'motivation', or 'expectancy' may play a central role in the relationship, then more emphasis should be placed on refining these concepts and some efforts should be made to measure their constituents. In this context, experience derived from other forms of psychotherapy should not be totally rejected, at least without being properly investigated.

2. Therapist's variables: The research on therapist's variables is disappointing, even with psychotherapies in which the therapeutic relationship plays a crucial role. In most cases we expect patients to use the therapist as a model, but at the same time we are not sure whether such modelling is limited only to therapist's approach

behaviours, or is extended to cover other characteristics as well. In addition, the precise nature of therapists' social reinforcing role has not been adequately investigated. Questions such as 'social reinforcement by whom, for which purpose, with which technique and under which conditions' have to be answered. In this context, therapist's identity merits further exploration. Furthermore, therapist's variables are obviously connected with training targets and selection criteria regarding patient–therapist–technique compatibility.

3. Communication variables: In the recent years experimental evidence has been accumulated regarding the effects of non-verbal communication (visual, postural etc.) on human attitude change. Most authors agree that non-verbal behaviour may serve a number of functions: expressive, monitoring, regulatory, and/or as related to personality and state of arousal. It is, therefore, suggested that a formal non-verbal analysis of videotaped behaviour therapy sessions might provide some useful information regarding patient–therapist relationship (Argyle, 1972; Patterson, 1976).

Finally, more weight should be given to a number of methodological issues, such as the developement of measuring instruments, the utilization of more 'single case' designs and the reliability of patients' and therapists' self-reports. Practical and theoretical difficulties do exist, but in our present state of knowledge, rejection of the therapeutic relationship as a target for further research could be counterproductive.

REFERENCES

Argyle, M. (1979) *The psychology of interpersonal behaviour.* Penguin Books, London.
Emmelkamp, P. M. G., and Kraanen, J. (1977) Therapist-controlled exposure *in vivo* vs self-controlled exposure *in vivo*: A comparison with obsessive–compulsive patients. *Behaviour Research and Therapy*, **15**, 491–495.
Eysenck, J. H. and Eysenck, B. G. S. (1964) *Manual of the Eysenck Personality Inventory.* University of London Press, London.
Fielder, F. E. (1950) The concept of an ideal therapeutic relationship. *Journal of Consulting Psychology*, **15**, 32–38.
Foa, E. B., and Steketee, G. S. (1979) Obsessive–compulsives: Conceptual issues and treatment interventions, in Hersen, M., Eisler, R. M., and Miller, P. M. (eds.) *Progress in Behaviour Modification*, Academic Press, New York, Vol. 8, pp. 1–53.
Gardner, G. G. (1964) The psychotherapeutic relationship. *Psychological Bulletin*, **61**, 426–437.
Gelder, M. G., Bancroft, J. H. S., Gath, D. H., Johnston, D. W., Mathews, A. M., and Shaw, P. M. (1973) Specific and non-specific factors in behaviour therapy. *British Journal of Psychiatry*, **123**, 445–462.
Goldstein, A. P., and Simonson, N. R. (1970) Social Psychological approaches to psychotherapy research, in Bergin, A. E. and Gafield, S. (eds.) *Handbook of Behaviour Changes in Children: A Pilot Study.* John Wiley, New York.
Goldstein, A. P., Heller, K., and Sechrest, L. B. (1966) *Psychotherapy and the psychology of behaviour change* John Wiley, New York.
Liberman, R. (1970) A Behavioural Approach to Group Dynamics. *Behaviour Therapy*, **1**, 312–327.

Mathews, A. M., (1977) Behavioural treatment of agoraphobia: New findings, new problems, in Boulougouris, J. C., and Rabavilas, A. D., (eds.) *The Treatment of Phobic and Obsessive–Compulsive Disorders* Pergamon Press, Oxford. pp. 1–5.

Mathews, A. M., Jonston, D. W., Lancashire, M., Munby, M., Shaw., P. M., and Gelder, M. G. (1976) Imagimal flooding and exposure to real phobic situations: Treatment outcome with agoraphobia patients. *British Journal of Psychiatry*, **129**, 362–371.

Patterson, M. L. (1976) An arousal model of interpersonal intimacy. *Psychological Review*, **83**, 235–245.

Rabavilas, A., Boulougouris, J. C., and Perissaki, C. (1979) Therapist qualities related to outcome with exposure *in vivo* in neurotic patients. *Journal of Behaviour Therapy and Experimental Psychiatry*, **10**, 293–294.

Schofield, W. (1969) *Psychotherapy, the Purchase of Friendship*. Prentice-Hall, Englewood Cliffs, New Jersey.

Spielberger, D. C., Gorsuch, R. L., and Lushene, E. R. (1970) *Manual for the State-Trait Anxiety Inventory*. Consulting Psychologists Press, Palo Alto, California.

Staats, A. W. (1964) *Human learning*. Holt, Rinehart & Winston, New York.

Sundland, D. H., and Barker, E. N. (1962) The orientation of psychotherapists. *Journal of Consulting Psychology*, **26**, 201–212.

Truax, C. B. (1961) *Therapeutic conditions*. University of Wisconsin Psychiatric Institute Bulletin, 1 (No. 10c).

Wilson, G. T., and Hannon, A. E. (1968) Behaviour therapy and the therapist–patient relationship. *Journal of Consulting Clinical Psychology*, **32**, 103–109.

IV. TREATMENT OF SEXUAL DISORDERS

Learning Theory Approaches to Psychiatry
Edited by John Boulougouris
© 1982 John Wiley & Sons Ltd

14. TREATMENT OF FEMALE SEXUAL DYSFUNCTION

Andrew Mathews

It is now a decade since the publication of *Human Sexual Inadequacy* (Masters and Johnson, 1970) and perhaps therefore a fitting time to re-evaluate our state of knowledge about sexual dysfunction. Clearly there has been a marked increase in enthusiasm and optimism about treatment results, but advances in our understanding of aetiology and treatment mechanism are less obvious. Although not always made explicit, there is a common assumption that dysfunction occurs when sexual responses are blocked by anxiety, and treatment involves removing this anxiety.

Progress in understanding the mechanism of other behavioural treatments has been made by use of the method of dismantling; dividing the complete procedure into its various components and testing their effectiveness. Within the procedure described by Masters and Johnson there seems to be at least two components; guided practice and sexual counselling. To compare the respective contributions of these two components would thus require three treatments, guided practice alone, counselling alone, and the two in combination. In designing a first study we felt it would be difficult to use counselling without giving any behavioural direction, and compromised by combining counselling with an alternative to Masters and Johnson's guided practice, imaginal desensitization. The three treatments compared by Mathews *et al.* (1976) were thus: (1) Imaginal desensitization with counselling, during weekly visits. (2) Instructions for directed practice with counselling. (3) Directed practice without counselling. The last requirement, that of witholding counselling, we felt was best accomplished by minimizing the actual contact between patients and therapist. This was reduced to three meetings during the twelve-week treatment period, and week-by-week directions for practice were sent by post. The other main factor in this design was whether or not couples were seen by one or two therapists.

Post-treatment ratings of sexual relationships gave indications of a marginal trend in favour of our fuller version of the Masters and Johnson procedure, most clearly so when two therapists were involved. However, this global effect tells us little about what behaviour actually changed. Considering only the couples in whom the woman was the main complainant, orgasmic failure and lack of sexual enjoyment seemed the most striking complaints, but treatment had virtually no effect on ratings of orgasmic response. On the other hand, ratings of enjoyment did change and followed the same trend as other results; that of better results following the guided practice with counselling.

The nature of the difficulties encountered in practice suggests that in the absence of the encouragement to discuss these difficulties openly during the weekly counselling sessions, couples are less likely to resolve them and continue. In the 'postal' treatment, some couples—particularly those with difficult marital relationships in general—simply come to a full stop when problems were encountered during practice, one or the other partner refusing to co-operate further.

The question of the nature of the change as perceived by the couples themselves was pursued using semantic differential ratings, collected before and after treatment. The semantic differentials included the adjectives used previously by Marks and Sartorius with sexually deviant patients, and also some new scales more appropriate to the present couples. Factor analyses with varimax rotation were completed for each sex and each occasion, and five factors selected that emerged consistently, defined as 'loving', 'anxious', 'attractive', 'good', and 'arousable'. Scores on each of these factors were then used to examine treatment effects as before. With these additional measures, on four out of five factors, S.D. scores for 'myself' changed significantly more in the practice plus counselling condition than in at least one of the other treatments, and more than both of the others in the case of 'attractive' and 'arousable' (Whitehead and Mathews, 1977).

Both men and women agreed in the S.D. ratings of 'arousability' that the women, especially if they were considered the main complainant of the couple, were harder to arouse than were the men. Although difficult to substantiate fully, because of the different dysfunctions involved, it did seem that lack of sexual response on the part of the woman was associated with poorer outcome than was (say) erectile impotence in the man.

Summarizing the results so far, it does not seem that the changes occurring in successful treatment fit any simple model of anxiety reduction. Directed practice with counselling produced more change than desensitization and the nature of the change reported by the couples themselves had more to do with increases in enjoyment and arousability than with anxiety reduction.

It remains possible, however, that these increases in arousal were secondary to a reduction of anxiety associated with sexual performance, brought about by the '*in vivo* exposure' element in guided practice. Alternatively a more general reduction in sexual anxiety might be relevant only on a subgroup of clients in whom the sexual dysfunction is of a phobic sort, while in others anxiety is less relevant.

In the second study (Carney *et al.*, 1978), we narrowed the range of presenting couples by selecting couples in whom the woman complained of lack of sexual responsiveness. In some of these women the problem seemed to present as a total lack of sexual interest or drive, while others complained of a definite aversion to sex, accompanied by anxiety, or similar negative feelings. Women given androgens for other medical reasons have been reported to experience an increase in sexual drive and interest, it was thought that those women with low interest might respond to androgens, while the more anxious women might be helped by tranquillizers. The main feature of the study design was thus the allocation of couples—who were all given some behavioural direction along the same lines as the earlier study—to either androgen therapy or a minor tranquillizer. The women were asked to take their medication (either active Testoral 10 mg and placebo Valium, or active Valium 10 mg and placebo Testoral) shortly before practice sessions or when going to bed. A further variable included in the design was the frequency of therapy sessions—weekly or monthly—to further investigate the importance of therapist contact and counselling.

Results did not entirely meet prediction, but were very clearcut. Over-all the group allocated to testosterone had a significantly better outcome than the group allocated to diazepam. This was a highly significant effect on the assessor's ratings of sexual relationship in a blind-study, although as indicated before, the improvement on this measure does not indicate very clearly what the nature of these changes were. The other measures showing a significant superiority for testosterone were almost all ratings by the women indicating an increase in the pleasant feelings associated with sexual activity. The best example is perhaps the increase in average rating of satisfaction for lovemaking, based on a detailed behavioural diary, in the absence of any significant change in the over-all amount of sexual contact. The women receiving testosterone (but not those having diazepam) also indicated an increase in the frequency of experiencing a climax. Semantic differential scores also favour the hormone group, but the effect was of the women rating the man as having changed more, with higher scores for the 'good', 'attractive', and 'loving' factors. A few semantic differential measures also show significant interaction between drugs and the 'high anxiety' or 'low drive' categorization of the woman. In every case this is the predicted direction, that is of diazepam apparently being more helpful with the 'high anxious' woman, and the hormone with 'low drive' women.

One set of significant effects which came as a complete surprise were those associated with treatment frequency—none favoured the high-frequency treatment, and a few even favoured the low-frequency condition. Since those measures showing this effect all related to ratings of anxiety in the male partner, one possible explanation is that husbands may have found their inability to satisfy their wives very threatening to their self-esteem, and that frequent sessions in which this was discussed may have made the resultant tension worse.

In a third study, which is continuing at present, we are attempting to re-examine some of the equivocal findings from research so far. These include the suggestion that two therapists (a dual-sex pair) may have a marginally better effect than one therapist alone, that there is no disadvantage to monthly as opposed to weekly treatments, and that psychological treatment effects may be enhanced by the simultaneous use of testosterone. Since these factors could interact, all combinations of one versus two therapists, monthly versus weekly sessions, and testosterone versus placebo were used in a factorial design. Treatment was offered to all couples seen in whom the main problem was lack of sexual responsiveness in the woman, after excluding those complaining only of orgasmic dysfunction, those with severe vaginismus, or of having a partner with erectile impotence. In practice the majority of female referrals met these requirements, although in the course of completing treatment with 36 couples, another 20 failed to complete, and seven were accepted but failed to start, giving the high drop-out rate of 43 %. Drop-outs were spread over conditions, although they tended to be more common during treatment by one rather than two therapists, and when there was a poor marital relationship.

Once accepted, couples were assigned at random to a single therapist or dual-sex pair, to either weekly or monthly visits, and to testosterone or matching placebo. Regular contact continued for just over three months, after which the couples were reassessed and followed up for six months.

Treatment procedures followed those used previously, based on our out-patient adaptation of Masters and Johnson's method. Despite excluding those complaining only of orgasmic dysfunction a total of 18 women out of the 36 included were not reaching orgasm by any means before treatment. In anticipation of this the treatment procedure used previously was made more flexible by incorporating some optional sets of instructions, one of which described techniques of female self-stimulation. Therapists discussed this with couples once mutual pleasuring sessions had begun, but did not insist on its use if this seemed unacceptable to the woman or her partner. Only in a minority of our couples did self-stimulation training seem both relevant and acceptable to both partners.

Analysis of the results from the first 36 couples showed that unexpectedly, none of the three factors varied appeared to be associated with differences in outcome. Considering first the drug effect, which seemed the most powerful in the previous study, none of the main outcome measures show any indication of differences (Table 1). Such a clear negative finding casts serious doubts on the earlier conclusion based on the comparison of testosterone with diazepam. Although the previous data had been interpreted as showing that testosterone had a positive effect, rather than the tranquillizers having a negative effect, the present results suggest that the latter

Table 1.   Sexual relations

	Pre-treatment	Post-treatment	Change
2 Therapists	4.0	2.6	1.4
1 Therapist	3.9	2.4	1.6
Weekly	3.9	2.3	1.6
Monthly	4.1	2.7	1.4
Testosterone	4.2	2.8	1.4
Placebo	3.7	2.2	1.5

Rating 1–5

explanation may have been the correct one. The corollary of this is that testosterone deficiency is not relevant to the aetiology of treatment of most female sexual dysfunctions. There is no indication of an interaction with other factors such that testosterone has more effect under some conditions of psychological treatment. This is not in fact surprising, since there is no evidence that any of the variations in treatment contact actually modified the effectiveness of treatment. The weekly versus monthly contact was originally seen as a way of assessing strong versus weak forms of psychological treatment; however, the differences in effectiveness are very small and unlikely to reach significance even with a much larger group of couples. Finally, the number of therapists also had little obvious effect on ratings of sexual function, although there is some indication that general marital relationship is slightly improved in the dual therapist condition only (Table 2).

Table 2.   General relations

	Pre-treatment	Post-treatment	Change
2 Therapists	2.5	1.9	0.6
1 Therapist	1.5	1.6	− 0.1
Weekly	1.8	1.7	0.1
Monthly	2.1	1.8	0.3
Testosterone	2.1	1.8	0.3
Placebo	1.8	1.6	0.2

Rating 1–5

A number of difficult questions are raised by this failure to find any convincing differences. Can we be certain that the treatments were equally effective, rather than equally ineffective? If they were effective, why are five sessions apparently just as good as 13 sessions? What if anything can we infer about the nature of female sexual dysfunction and the mechanisms of treatment?

We can be reasonably certain that our treatment was effective. The over-all change achieved on the present trial on the assessors ratings of sexual relationship was one and a half points on the 1–5 scale. This is almost the same as was achieved in the best treatment condition within our first trial, and similarly identical to the change achieved by the group receiving testosterone in the second trial. In fact the only group at odds with the rest is those who had been given diazepam, who showed only about half the magnitude of over-all change (0.7 points on the 1–5 scale). This would seem to add strong support to the conclusion that rather than testosterone enhancing outcome, the tranquilliser actually reduced treatment effectiveness.

Apart from our own studies there are at least two others which have found similar treatment methods to be significantly better than a waiting list control group (Munjack et al., 1976; Dow, 1980). The latter study was particularly convincing in that the treatments replicated both our weekly out-patient modification of Masters and Johnson and a self-help group with written instructions and minimal contact. Both of these treatments were better than the wait group, while treatment with therapist counselling was better than the self-help condition only in couples having female loss of interest as the main problem. Thus, as with our own earlier study, self-help treatments with virtually no therapist contact are less effective with female problems in particular. This group characterized by loss of sexual interest, was also found to differ from others before treatment in having greater marital and communication problems. Combined with the present results this indicates that some therapist contact is necessary to treat the majority of these problems, but a large number of therapy sessions does not necessarily result in a greater effect. Giving practice instructions with virtually no therapist contact or counselling, is presumably ineffective because the difficulties in marital relationship and communication may quickly lead to a breakdown of co-operation in carrying out practice instructions. Occasional therapist contact is thus seen as necessary in order to find ways round these obstacles which would otherwise prevent further progress.

The present data show no obvious role for the dual therapist team, except perhaps in cases where the main obstacles to progress arise from severe marital conflict. At first glance, however, it is puzzling that the trend for two therapists to produce more improvement in marital relationship is not paralleled by a greater improvement in sexual relationships. A possible explanation may lie in the high drop-out rate already mentioned, as this seemed particularly acute with conflicted couples assigned to a single therapist. Thus the lack of a clear difference in favour of two therapists may be partly attributable to their greater success with keeping difficult couples in treatment.

Although a clear understanding of either aetiology or treatment mechanism is still elusive, the results of the studies described here may allow us to eliminate some of the less tenable theories. In particular the evidence against a simple anxiety reduction hypothesis of treatment is becoming increasingly compelling. Desensitization is relatively ineffective, anxiety measures change less than do ratings of enjoyment and arousal, and the use of anxiolytic medication appears to be counter-productive. None of these findings is conclusive, nor do they rule out a more specific role for anxiety at some stage in the development of some sexual difficulties, but they do suggest that other psychological processes must be involved. This view is further supported by recent laboratory findings that anxiety-evoking stimuli do not always inhibit sexual responding—indeed they may actually enhance sexual response under some circumstances (Hoon et al., 1977). Instead of being concerned with anxiety reduction, it would seem that we need to identify more precisely what psychological states or interpersonal behaviours can interfere with normal sexual responding. In many women these may be related to boredom, depression, resentment, or general dissatisfaction with partners; indicating a need to change some aspects of the marital situation. In others, who describe an otherwise excellent marital relationship, treatment may need to focus on ways of increasing interest and enjoyment. Although we incorporated a self-stimulation component in the most recent study, achieving orgasm by this method does not seem acceptable or relevant in many of our cases. For example, six women among the 36 were regularly orgasmic before treatment, but despite this reported little sexual interest or satisfaction. Observations such as these suggest that we need to look elsewhere to understand and treat the loss of sexual interest in these women.

REFERENCES

Carney, A., Bancroft, J., and Mathews, A. (1978) Combination of hormonal and psychological treatment for female sexual unresponsiveness: a comparative study. *British Journal of Psychiatry*, **133**, 339–346.

Dow, M. (1980) *A comparative evaluation of 'self-help' and conventional Masters and Johnson approaches for sexual dysfunction.* Paper delivered at the BABP conference, Aberdeen.

Hoon, P., Wincze, J., and Hoon, E. (1977) A test of reciprocal inhibition: are anxiety and sexual arousal in women mutually inhibitory? *Journal of Abnormal Psychology*, **86**, 65–74.

Masters, W., and Johnson, V. (1970) *Human Sexual Inadequacy*, Churchill, London.

Mathews, A., Bancroft, J., Whitehead, A., Hackman, A., Julien, D., Bancroft, J., Gath, D., and Shaw, P. (1976) The behavioural treatment of sexual inadequacy: a comparative study. *Behaviour Research and Therapy*, **14** 427–436.

Munjack, D., Cristol, A., Goldstein, A., Phillips, D., Goldberg, A., Whipple, K., Staples, F., and Kanno, P. (1976) Behavioural treatment of orgasmic dysfunction: a controlled study. *British Journal of Psychiatry*, **129**, 349–353.

Whitehead, A., and Mathews, A. (1977) Attitude change during behavioural treatment of sexual inadequacy. *British Journal of Social and Clinical Psychology*, **16**, 275–281.

Learning Theory Approaches to Psychiatry
Edited by John Boulougouris
© 1982 John Wiley & Sons Ltd

15. CURRENT RESEARCH ON SEXUAL DYSFUNCTION

Walter Everaerd

Since 1972, we have studied various approaches to the treatment of sexual dysfunction. Recently we began to follow up patients treated between 1972 and 1975 and contacted 120 couples though the response up to now has been small. Some were still enthusiastic about the therapy which they had received five or more years ago when satisfaction from their sexual interactions had increased and are still very positive. Negative evaluations were also found. Some couples had relapsed and others were seeking treatment again.

Although it is difficult to derive any definite conclusions from this follow-up, it is speculated that the results obtained from couples complaining about dysfunction in the male are less favourable. As early as 1975, it became quite clear that specific approaches had to be devised at least for some male complaints. Until then, treatment effects were very unsatisfactory. This study was started in order to deal with special difficulties of male sexual dysfunction and this chapter reports on the progress of this on-going project.

It seems to be the general opinion that male sexual complaints are a result of their performance orientation as opposed to feeling orientation. Inhibition and 'holding back' are often described as causative behaviours (Masters and Johnson, 1970; Kaplan, 1974). As often indicated in the literature, the analyses of ejaculatory difficulties supposed different coping behaviours for premature, retarded, and deficient ejaculation. Males suffering from premature ejaculation are essentially anxious, quickly withdraw from their feelings, and have especially short sexual interactions with their partners. For example one man, who was always premature *vis-à-vis* his wife, could control his ejaculatory response when entering her from the rear. By doing this, he probably avoided any emotional interaction.

Many males suffering from retarded or deficient ejaculation are sexually very effective with their partners who sometimes have multiple orgasms but who also often complain of lack of commitment on the part of their male partners. A number of males were 'untouchable'. They avoided every stimulating type of touch from their partners which could possibly result in a display of feeling.

Differentiation on psychological characteristics between male complaints has been attempted by Derogatis (1976) and Derogatis and Meyer (1979) and by Munjack *et al.* (1978). Using masculinity and femininity scales, Derogatis found dysfunctionals to have somewhat low scores on both dimensions. Male dysfunctionals tended to score higher on masculinity than femininity while female dysfunctionals tended to score lower on both dimensions compared with 'normals', i.e. non-dysfunctionals. Munjack and his colleagues (1978) found a significant difference between retarded and premature ejaculators. Retarded ejaculators had higher masculinity scores and similar differences were found by us. In Figure 1, masculinity scores are represented for different complaint groups. It seems that different complaints correlate with different coping styles. Premature ejaculators are coping with threats in sexual interactions by avoiding intimate interaction. Retarded ejaculators on the contrary often engage in intimate interactions with their partners but control the situation by being very active towards their partners. Their approach behaviour represents their way of coping with threats in such interaction.

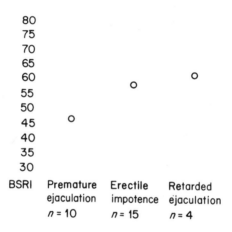

Figure 1.   Bem Sex Role Inventory—masculinity scores and male dysfunctions

Sex therapy aims at reducing avoidance of sexual interactions and sexual stimulation. Patients coping with approach behaviour are typically not avoiding interactions but defend themselves against any emotional involvement. To change these defences, we devised an approach by slightly modifying the Rational Emotive Therapy (Ellis, 1974). This on-going study compares sex therapy to modified RET (Table 1). While still gathering data based on this project, at the same time the RET approach to groups of males without partners or with partners who were not available for therapy (Everaerd *et al.*, 1981) is being applied. Up to now we have been able to evaluate a group format for five consecutive groups. Not only heterosexual males but also homosexuals were admitted to these groups. During the intake procedure, the group synthesis was discussed with each applicant and there was no objection to such group composition. Although 47 men applied for the

Table 1. Design: Treatment of male dysfunctions in couples

	Sex therapy	RET
Premature ejaculation: Actual or in history	success predicted	
Erectile impotence and Retarded ejaculation		success predicted

programme, only 27 took part in one of the groups. Finally, 21 males, four exclusively homosexual, three mixed homo-heterosexual, and 14 exclusively heterosexual completed the programme. Drop-outs during or even before intake are represented in Table 2. Six dropped out during therapy, two due to lack of motivation and four for reasons associated with the nature of the programme. These reasons varied from an inconvenient time-schedule to strong emotional reactions which were unmanageable in the group. The latter four men were treated individually.

Table 2. Reasons and number of drop-outs

Total number of applicants	47
Did not appear for intake	5
Stayed away after intake	8
Came into therapy with a partner	2
Referred elsewhere in connection:	
With non-sexual complaint	2
Underwent still another therapy	2
Somatic complaint	1
Total number of drop-outs before therapy	20
Number of clients in therapy	27
Drop-outs during therapy	6
Number of clients completed therapy	21

The group method was structured into three consecutive blocks. (Table 3). RET was used to make it clear to patients that they themselves can realize the conditions for arousal and help the clients to reinterpret their bodily sensations if necessary. The method served also to change, on a cognitive level, fear of failure, spectatoring, and negative self-image as a result of sexual dysfunction. Patients made an analysis at home whenever they experienced difficulties with their sexuality. They also used imagery exercises to practise new behaviour in fantasy.

Table 3. Procedure of group method sessions

Intake   group (15–20 sessions)
Block 1: 5 sessions RET adaptation
Block 2: 5 sessions sensate focus + masturbation
Block 3: 5 sessions social skills in relation to sexuality

Sessions aimed at sensate focus and masturbation were used to direct attention to bodily and sexual feelings. Special attention was given to non-genital sensations. Specific instructions were used for different complaints, i.e. Seman's stop–start method (Semans, 1956) with premature ejaculation; teasing with erectile impotence; successive approximation with retarded or deficient ejaculation. In the last block of sessions the attention was focused on social skills related to sexuality. After analysing difficult situations with the help of RET, patients role-played new behaviour in the group. Each group had two male therapists who were trained and experienced in sex therapy for couples.

Evaluation of the effects of the programme consisted of patients' subjective account of their sexual functioning and of psychometric tests.

The subjective account consisted of:
1. Diary with three standardized questions:
    (a) What did you get out of the last session?
    (b) What are you going to do with this information?
    (c) What have you done this week?
2. At the termination of therapy an extensive evaluation was written concerning changes especially in sexual functioning.
3. At two months follow up an interview on sexual functioning.

The psychometric tests were:
1. The Sexuality Experience Scales (Frenken, 1976) and an adapted version for homosexual patients.
2. Willems Social Anxiety Scale (Willems et al., 1973).
3. Bem's Sex Role Inventory (Bem, 1974).

The results of treatment in groups are represented in Table 4. In this Table change of dysfunction is specified for two stimulation conditions e.g. masturbation and interaction with a partner. Some patients had no interactions with partners. Success was also rated independently by patients and therapists on a three-point rating scale. Ratings of both patients and therapists strongly agree with change in sexual dysfunction. At follow-up, two months after completing therapy, the post-treatment results were confirmed. Those who had most improved (+ +) and those who were not changed at all (O O) still functioned at that same level. Some improvement was seen in some of the patients who failed with a partner or had no partner during therapy.

The results on the psychometric tests were unsatisfactory. Mainly because the measurement area of the Sexuality Experience Scales does not fully overlap with the goals of the group method. Although this scale is strongly based in favour of coitus orgasm we did find significant differences between pre- and post-treatment comparisons. However, comparable studies have not been done on a large scale. Some of the studies show results resembling ours. Zilbergeld (1975) reported that:

Table 4. Number of clients showing changes in sexual dysfunction and clients' and therapists' success ratings

| Dysfunction | Change in dysfunction | | | | | Success-ratings | | | | | |
| | | | | | | Client | | | Therapist | | |
	+ +	+ ?	+ O	O ?	O O	2	1	0	2	1	0
Premature ejaculation (n = 7)	1	2	3	1	0	2	3	2	1	5	1
Erectile impotence (n = 10)	5	3	0	1	1	6	2	2	5	3	2
Retarded ejaculation (n = 4)	2	1	1	0	0	3	1	0	4	0	0

+ + = during masturbation and with partner
+ ? = during masturbation, no partner experience
+ O = during masturbation, but *not* with partner
O ? = *not* during masturbation, no partner experience
O O = *not* during masturbation, *not* with partner

2 = high
1 = average
0 = low

'two-thirds of his patients felt they had completely achieved their goals by the end of therapy'. He is, however, not clear about the criteria for success. Zeiss *et al.* (1978) reported noticeable progress in four out of six cases. At follow-up one of the four seemed to have relapsed. Lobitz and Baker (1979) reported that six out of nine patients recorded noticeable improvement. In three cases no data are furnished seeing that the clients had no new coitus experience. At follow-up two of the six patients appeared to be completely cured.

In view of results obtained by others, we can consider our programme reasonably successful. A comparison of our results with other studies is hampered by the fact that in other studies the changes in sexual dysfunction by means of masturbation has not been evaluated. In conjunction with our results, it should be noted that 16 of the 21 patients came into therapy with primary complaints. At the same time, the average and median duration of the complaints were respectively six and four years. Looking back at our experiences with the groups a weak point in using our programme is indicated. Males complaining of premature ejaculation did not improve as much as males with other complaints. This might be attributed to the general nature of interventions as used in the programme. These were aimed at attacking and reducing defensive behaviours of the approach type. We can also speculate that the block of sessions aimed at social skills training was not adequately structured so as to help these males in their interactions. The on-going study with couples might give us some clues as to the significance of the interaction between complaint and therapy-method.

To conclude, I would like to stress a difficult point in managing male patients. In Table 1 it was shown how many drop-outs occurred from intake to therapy. Accepting any assistance seems to be very difficult for many males. Besides the defence that this attitude implicates, it also implies a certain conception of sexual motivation. In the sexological literature there appears to be a general awareness of this problem. Recently Kolodny *et al.* (1979) and Kaplan (1979) wrote about low sexual desire and sexual aversion. These texts specify some very general negative expectations and consequences of negative sexual experiences. But at the same time they show how poorly sexual motivation is understood. It seems that social control over sexual behaviour is not so easily uncovered. In the therapy of sexual dysfunction, patients are helped to define what sexuality is. Some years ago sex was mainly seen as coitus and orgasm through coital stimulation. Now, it seems, feeling is very dominant in defining sex. Undoubtedly there will be new definitions. These definitions, although propagated with pleasurable promises, take control over the lives of many people. Most therapists are as much under the control of these various definitions as are their patients. Therapists seem to know what sex is, but like their patients they do not know why they themselves behave sexually. 'Yes,' said one patient, 'I am not a machine, so I cannot ask why it does not work, I will have to turn the question upside down, why am I not a machine?'

REFERENCES

Bem, S. L. (1974) The measurement of psychological androgyny. *Journal of Consulting Clinical Psychology*, **42**, 155–162.

Derogatis, L. R. (1976) Psychological assessment of sexual disorders, in Meyer, J. K. (ed.) *Clinical Management of sexual disorders*. The Williams and Wilkins Company, Baltimore, pp. 35–73.

Derogatis, L. R., and Meyer, J. K. (1979) A psychological profile of the sexual dysfunctions. *Archives of Sexual Behavior*, **8**, 201–223.

Ellis, A. (1974) *Humanistic Psychotherapy*, McGraw, New York.

Everaerd, W., Dekker, J., Dronkers, J., van Rhee, K., Staffeleu, J., and Wiselius, G. (1981) Treatment of sexual dysfunction in male-only groups. (submitted for publication).

Frenken, J. (1976) *Afkeer van sexualiteit*, Van Loghum Slaterus, Deventer.

Kaplan, H. S. (1974) *The new sex therapy*, Brunner-Mazel, New York.

Kaplan, H. S. (1979) *Problems of sexual desire*. Brunner-Mazel, New York.

Kolodny, R. C., Masters, W. H., and Johnson, V. E. (1979) *Textbook of Sexual Medicine*, Little, Brown, Boston.

Lobitz, W. C., and Baker, E. L. (1979) Group treatment of single males with erectile dysfunction. *Archives of Sexual Behavior*, **8**, 127–138.

Masters, W. H., and Johnson, V. E. (1970) *Human Sexual Inadequacy*, Churchill, London.

Munjack, D., Kanno, P., and Oziel, L. (1978) Ejaculatory disorders: Some psychometric data. *Psychological Reports*, **43**, 783–787.

Semans, J. (1956) Premature Ejaculation, a new approach. *South Medical Journal*, **49**, 353–358.

Willems, L. F. M., Tuender-de Haan, H. A., and de Fares, P. B. (1973) Een schaal om sociale angst te meten. *Nederlands Tijdschrift voor Psychologie*, **28**, 415–422.

Zilbergeld, B. (1975) Group treatment of sexual dysfunction in men without partner. *Journal of Sex and Marital Therapy*, **1**, 204–214.

Zeiss, R. A., Christensen, A., and Levine, A. G. (1978) Treatment for premature ejaculation through male-only groups. *Journal of Sex and Marital Therapy*, **4**, 139–143.

Learning Theory Approaches to Psychiatry
Edited by John Boulougouris
© 1982 John Wiley & Sons Ltd

16. BEHAVIOUR THERAPY IN GROUPS OF PATIENTS WITHOUT PARTNERS AND COUPLES SUFFERING FROM SEXUAL DYSFUNCTION

Götz Kockott

This chapter gives a preliminary report of an on-going project in which therapy for individual patients with sexual dysfunction is being examined. The project design, the results, and the experiences in dealing with these patient-groups will be discussed. The effectiveness of the Masters and Johnson method and its variations in the treatment of couples suffering from sexual dysfunction is well-established. Recently, treatment of three to four couples in a group has been described as a successful method as well. There are, however, no therapeutic programmes available for individual patients suffering from sexual inadequacy except masturbation training in groups for preorgasmic women (Barbach, 1974) and treatment of sociosexual anxieties in groups for men (Arentewicz et al., 1978).

Thus, the reason for this study, in which individual patients are treated together with couples in a mixed sex group, is that it is believed that individual patients may benefit from the presence of couples for the following reasons. First, patients gain the opportunity of imitation learning and second, patients participate in a communication setting, which facilitates treatment directed towards their sexual problems.

The subjects are patients suffering from psychogenic erectile impotence or from orgasmic dysfunction. Individual patients were selected who had experienced their sexual problems in more than one partnership so that partner-dependent sexual problems were ruled out. Patients with a severely disturbed partnership, schizoid patients who were extremely handicapped in their ability to form a partnership, and patients with psychotic symptomatology were excluded using a semistructured psychiatric interview.

The subjects were assigned arbitrarily to one of the following three groups (Table 1): The first group consists of couples only. The second group consists of individual patients only i.e. four male and four female patients. The third group consists of couples and individual patients i.e. two couples, two male, and two female patients.

Table 1.   Therapy design

	Couple group	Individual group	Mixed group
Treatment groups	Four couples	Four female, four male individual patients	Two couples and two female, two male
Treatment schedule	Behaviourally oriented. Initially three sessions in one day, 12–15 weekly sessions, one booster session every six weeks up to a total of four		
Treatment results	Pre- and post-treatment comparison and follow-up a. semistructured interview b. diaries c. set of questionnaires		

There is also a waiting list group of couples and individual patients who will later be assigned to one of the above kind of therapy groups.

Each group is treated by two therapists with an initial phase of three sessions in one day followed by approximately 12–15 weekly sessions and followed by one booster session every six weeks up to a total of four. The initial phase is thought to increase group cohesion. At least three pre-sessions are used for behaviour analysis. The therapeutic success is being measured by means of a pre- and post-treatment comparison and follow-up using the following testings: (1) semistructured interview focused on sexual symptomatology; (2) diaries kept by the patients during the 14 days before and the last 14 days of therapy focusing on sexual behaviour and sexual social anxieties; and (3) battery of questionnaires: i.e. FPI personality questionnaire (Fahrenberg *et al.*, 1973); questionnaire about self-assertion (Ullrich and Ullrich-de Muynck, 1976); questionnaire relating to attitude towards one's own body (EKM); sexual anxiety questionnaire (Dittmar *et al.*, 1977) and a Sexual Interaction Inventory (LoPiccolo, 1974).

The therapy is mainly behaviourally orientated, using the methods of Masters and Johnson (1970), LoPiccolo and Lobitz (1972), masturbation training for women and Zilbergeld (1978), masturbation training for erectile impotence, slightly modified. Treatment also includes sex education, communication training, and role playing. Each session is constructed approximately as follows (Table 2):

1. Short self-reports as understood in Gestalt therapy: each group member states how he feels at that moment and whether he has any specific problems at that particular moment.
2. Short discussion of current problems and discussion about the tasks given to all members as 'homework'.
3. Discussion of specific home tasks in so-called mini-groups—both the therapists discuss the experiences of these tasks with half of the group which is sometimes sex specific (male/female) and sometimes problem specific (erectile/orgasmic disturbance).

4. A specific topic is worked on by the whole group by means of discussion, specific communication exercises, role playing etc. Such topics are: information about sexual dysfunction, relationship training, sexual anxieties, sexual avoidance behaviour, body contact, communication rules, masturbation, how to express wishes, how to express sexual wishes, how to handle conflicts, simulation of disorder occurrence, and rehearsal of solutions in such a situation (Zilbergeld, 1978).
5. Short self-reports (as (1) above).

Table 2.   Structure of the group sessions

1. Self-report of present state
2. Group discussion of tasks carried out at home
3. In mini-groups: discussion of specific tasks
4. In the group: working on a specific topic
5. Self-report of present state

RESULTS

Intermediate

Mixed group This pilot-study group, a mixed group of two couples and four individual patients was constructed in order to observe the possibility of treating couples and individual patients together in one group. Selection was not carefully carried out and patients were included in the group who should not have been. Two individual patients had been alcoholics, one had an ejaculatory incompetence and one couple had a rather disturbed relationship.

In summary the results were as follows. One couple improved remarkably i.e. the husband lost his erectile impotence. The other couple had to be sent to partnertherapy. One individual patient, who had been alcoholic, built up a partnership free of sexual dysfunction. There was no change in the sexual problem of the individual who suffered from ejaculatory incompetence but he became much more self-assertive. One female individual patient, who had also been an alcoholic, improved her attitude towards her own body, but was still afraid to engage in sexual contact. Finally, one female individual patient discontinued therapy after the tenth session and joined a sensitivity-training group without a therapist.

Couple group Within the main project, we have completed the programme with one couple group. A short description and the results of this couple group will be discussed in more detail. The whole group consisted of four couples. Two male patients suffered from primary erectile impotence and two female patients from primary complete anorgasmia. All patients had partners. The age range was between 20 years and 32 years. The partnerships had already lasted from six months to five years. One couple was married and had a two-year-old son. All members were middle-class, their occupations being clerk, housewife, nurse, student. Two couples were referred by their gynaecologist, two came on their own initiative.

The data derived from the semistandardized interviews are as follows. Couple one. The man was suffering from primary erectile impotence which made sexual intercourse impossible, the female partner had no sexual disturbances. At the end of therapy both were satisfied with their sexual activity as compared to pre-therapy dissatisfaction. Erections occurred during petting and superficial intromission was possible. Anxiety feelings during sexual contact, which appeared most of the time before therapy, almost disappeared and there was no longer any sexual avoidance behaviour. There were no changes in the undisturbed sexual behaviour of the female partner.

Couple two. This couple shows a rather similar picture: the man before therapy suffered from primary erectile impotence which made sexual intercourse impossible. The female partner was slightly inhibited sexually but did not show any overt sexual disturbance. At the end of therapy both partners were satisfied with their sexual activity as compared to the pre-therapy dissatisfaction; erections occurred during petting and superficial intromission was possible; anxiety feelings during sexual contact and sexual avoidance behaviour had decreased from 'always present' to 'only sometimes present'. There were no changes in the undisturbed sexual behaviour of the female partner.

Couple three. Before therapy started, the woman was completely anorgasmic while the man had slight erectile difficulties. During the time of assessment before therapy the sexual avoidance behaviour of the female had already decreased so much that at the beginning of therapy both were satisfied with their sexual activity to a certain degree, but the woman was still anorgasmic. At the end of therapy, the woman experienced orgasm while masturbating and masturbated approximately once a week; lubrication increased during petting; positive feelings during coitus increased substantially; sexual avoidance behaviour disappeared completely and she was orgasmic during coitus when also using a vibrator. The male partner lost his occasional sexual anxiety feelings and did not experience any erectile difficulties anymore.

Couple four. Before therapy the woman was anorgasmic and had never masturbated. The husband had a tendency to ejaculate prematurely. At the end of therapy both were satisfied with their sexual activity as compared to complete dissatisfaction before. The wife had learned to masturbate more than once a week, enjoyed it, and had orgasm. Lubrication increased during petting and coitus; positive feelings increased and she experienced orgasm during petting by manual stimulation by her husband but not yet during coitus. The husband's tendency for premature ejaculation has not changed so far.

No changes in any couple were reflected in the administered general questionnaires such as personality questionnaire (FPI) and questionnaire about self-assertion. But there were some changes in the answers to specific questionnaires which shall be discussed with the follow-up results.

Follow-up

Mixed group In summary the patients' conditions four months after the end of intensive therapy can be described as follows: no relapse but also no further improvement in the patients.

Couple group Six months follow-up has been completed recently. The data derived from the semistandardized interviews are as follows:

Couple one. No longer any abnormal sexual symptoms. The couple is very satisfied with its sexual activity and partnership. Have since married.

Couple two. No more erectile disturbances; no sexual anxiety; no sexual avoidance behaviour. The couple is very satisfied with its sexual activity, has few partnership difficulties and became very active in social activities.

Couple three. Partners are both satisfied sexually and with their partnership. During coitus, the woman is orgasmic when simultaneous manual stimulation is used.

Couple four. The woman is very sexually satisfied and reaches orgasm during coitus using simultaneous manual stimulation. Husband's tendency to ejaculate prematurely has decreased. The couple has learned to handle its additional partner's problems much better.

The changes obtained from filling out the questionnaires are presented in Table 3. No changes were reflected either in the personality questionnaire (FPI) or in the questionnaire about self-assertion (U).

The questionnaire about attitude towards masturbation and towards one's own body, which was developed by our team of therapists, showed in three patients and two of their partners a marked change in attitude towards masturbation, which they can now accept as one form of sexual activity. One patient showed a positive change

Table 3. Couple group: Positive changes obtained on the questionnaires at six months follow-up

	EKM	Sexual attitude	Sexual anxiety	LoPiccolo inventory
Patient 1. (erectile impotence)	+ +			+
Patient 2. (erectile impotence)	+		+ +	+ +
Patient 3. (anorgasmia)	+ +	+		+
Patient 4. (anorgasmia)	+ +	+ +	+	+
Partner 1			+	+
Partner 2	+ +		+	+
Partner 3	+	+	+	+
Partner 4		+		+ +

+ = marked changes
+ + = very marked changes

in attitude towards her own body. The sexual attitude testing showed that both female patients and their partners decreased their conservatism towards sexuality. The sexual anxiety scale showed a clear decrease of anxiety in two patients and three partners. The scores on Sexual Interaction Inventory showed mild to marked improvement in all couples.

In general, all changes in specific questionnaires could be seen at the end of the intensive therapy and became more pronounced at the six months follow-up. In particular, changes in the partners of our patients are of special interest.

EXPERIENCES DEALING WITH PATIENT GROUPS

First, some remarks on the design of our project, second, on the content of treatment and third, on problems of standardization between groups. Regarding the design, care has to be taken in the selection of individual patients. This therapy does not seem to be useful for very schizoid patients who are severely handicapped in their ability to form a partnership. Round-table discussions with the couples before starting therapy are very important to clarify the symptomatology. At the same time, therapists can get a very good impression about the quality of the partnership. The pre-sessions themselves acquire therapeutic value. One couple improved so much during this time that no further therapy was needed. Therefore, it may be necessary to change our pre- and post-treatment comparison into a three-point comparison to establish therapeutic success; first point at the first pre-session, second point at the beginning, and third point at the end of therapy. However, even the patients' decision to undergo therapy is of therapeutic value but this is a difficult point to measure.

Groups of ten persons (two therapists and eight patients) are rather large. Smaller groups may be better but this causes a problem in the mixed group since arrangements such as one couple and four individual patients or two couples and two individual patients seem to disturb the equilibrium. We can agree with the impression held by different therapists that patients are more active in a treatment programme when the number of sessions are limited. After 12–15 weekly sessions, there seems to be a need by patients and therapists for a break. From then on, patients seem able to handle the rest of their sexual problems by themselves but ask for booster sessions.

As regards the content of therapy, sex education is still very important for patients with sexual dysfunction, even for the young ones. For instance, many women still find the acceptance of masturbation and clitoridal orgasm a big problem. Relaxation training was a help in therapy. Patients easily reached this first goal of the treatment programme and received reinforcement from it for continuing therapy and at the same time, they learned to become more aware of their bodies. Relaxation training was later used for treating specific problems such as erectile and orgasmic dysfunction. The simulation of disorder occurrence and rehearsal of solutions in such a situation was of great importance. The method of Zilbergeld was used, which is strongly recommended. Group interaction was very low and the main interaction took place between therapists and patients but not among patients themselves. Maybe this was due to the form of therapy. It still remains unclear how this influences therapy success. Another problem arose when some individual patients formed partnerships and were not prepared to tell their new partners that they were undergoing therapy. They were advised to inform their partners and were offered an interview together with their new partner outside the treatment programme but it was decided not to take the new partner into the on-going treatment.

Finally, standardization, especially regarding the content of therapy, is needed since differences may arise from the therapists having different professional backgrounds. Differences may also arise from the type of group as some tasks cannot be the same for couples and for individual patients. Different group compositions such as age and the duration of partnership seem to be two very important variables. Therefore, careful matching for these two variables is necessary.

We have assembled an extensive therapy manual guide for therapists with compulsory and optional instructions. With this approach, we hope to minimize the differences in therapy content although they cannot be completely avoided. For this reason, we have also planned rotation of the therapists among group types. In summary, therapy for sexual problems in groups of couples is possible but it remains to be seen which type of group shows the best results.

REFERENCES

Arentewicz, G., Bulla, K., Schoof-Tams, and Schorsch, E. (1975) Verhaltenstherapie sexueller Funktionsstörungen: Erfahrungen mit 23 Paaren, in Schorsch, E., and Schmidt, G. (eds.) *Ergebnisse zur Sexualforschung*, Kiepenheuer u. Witsch, Cologne.

Arentewicz, G., Höflich, B. and Eck, D. (1978) Therapie soziosexueller Ängste von Männern. *Sexualmedizin*, **1978** 639–644.

Barbach, L. G. (1974) Group treatment of preorgasmic women *Journal of Sexual and Marital Therapy*, **1**, 139–145.

Dittmar, F., Kockott, G., and Nusselt, L. (1977) Ein einfaches Instrument zur Messung von Gefühlen, angewendet als Kriterium des Therapieerfolges bei Erektionsstörungen, in Kockott, G. (ed.) *Sexuelle Störungen*, Urban & Schwarzenberg, Munich, Vienna, Baltimore.

Fahrenberg, J., Selg, H., and Hampel, R. (1973) *Freiburger Persönlickeitsinventar*, Hogrefe, Göttingen.

LoPiccolo, J. (1974) The sexual interaction inventory: a new instrument for assessment of sexual dysfunction *Archives of Sexual Behaviour*, **3**, 585–595.

LoPiccolo, J., and Lobitz, W. (1972) The role of masturbation in the treatment of orgasmic dysfunction. *Archives of Sexual Behaviour*, **2**, 163–171.

Masters, W. H., and Johnson, V. E. (1970) *Human sexual inadequacy*, Little, Brown, Boston.

Ullrich, R., and Ullrich-de Muynck, R. (1976) *Einübung von Selbstvertrauen and sozialer Kompetenz*, Pfeiffer, Munich.

Zilbergeld, B. (1978) *Male sexuality*, Little, Brown, Boston-Toronto.

Learning Theory Approaches to Psychiatry
Edited by John Boulougouris
© 1981 John Wiley & Sons Ltd

17. COUPLE THERAPY WITH PSYCHIATRIC PATIENTS

Friedemann Pfäfflin

When developing a new method of psychotherapeutic treatment it is advisable to define the patient's condition prior to therapy, the criteria of success as precisely as possible, and to keep a safe distance from disturbing factors by making a strict selection of patients. The success or failure of a method can be assessed with more certainty if the symptom can be clearly isolated, and therefore treatment is concentrated more on the one sympton in question. The method of treating sexual dysfunctions introduced by Masters and Johnson (1970) appears to meet these requirements almost ideally, precisely defining sexual dysfunctions which, it seems, often appear in isolation. The successful treatment outcome can be operationalized and the rate of success is unusually high.

However, on closer examination of the publications of Masters and Johnson and of second and third generation therapists who orient their work on this method, one notices a conspicuous general lack of precision in the descriptions of patient samples, the therapeutic procedure and the operationalizing of successful treatment. On the other hand, the tendency for patients to be refused admittance to the treatment programme if they show signs, besides sexual dysfunctions, of pathological or other dysfunctions, is unmistakable. LoPiccolo and Lobitz (1973), for example, excluded nearly every second couple from treatment, basing their decision on a short interview, a test using the MMPI for exclusion of subclinical psychosis, and the Locke–Wallace–Short Marital Inventory for exclusion of seriously disrupted relationships. Other research teams rely on different methods by, for example, using psychological tests for neuroses as selection criteria. What is involved in each case are the research group's preliminary decisions, which can at the most be described as coincidental, as to which patients are to be treated and which not. Or is it perhaps a conceptional problem and not just a coincidence that almost all so-called seriously disturbed personalities or couples and all psychiatrically conspicuous couples are excluded?

In the following section the problem of indication for couple therapy will be clarified a little further. With particular reference to psychiatric patients, some data taken from a research project carried out in Hamburg will first be mentioned and then an outline of the case histories of three couples with psychiatric dysfunctions. To conclude, a few theses for future research have been formulated.

179

AIMS AND RESULTS OF THE RESEARCH PROJECT

Between 1972 and 1979, 262 couples with chronic sexual dysfunctions (90% for more than three years; 10% for more than six years) were treated at the Department of Sex Research. The research project had two main aims:

1. To adapt the models developed by Masters and Johnson to German conditions.
2. To test whether modified settings are just as effective as intensive therapy with two therapists.

   These aims were summarized as follows. We wished to shape the method of treatment, which the results of Masters and Johnson had clearly shown to be successful, into a form of treatment available to as many strata of society as possible, at the smallest possible expense. Selection of couples was made according to purely general and formal criteria. Both partners should show a basic desire to continue the relationship; should not engage in any external sexual relationships during treatment, and should not be in treatment elsewhere. Contraceptive precautions should be taken. Severe dependence on alcohol or drugs and psychosis in the acute stage when in-patient treatment was necessary were judged to be factors that invalidate indication.

   The 262 couples were treated by 29 therapists in the following settings:

1. Intensive therapy with two therapists: Male and female therapists formed a therapists' team. Daily sessions six times a week were held for three weeks, making a total of 18 therapy sessions, including individual in depth discussions between each therapist and patient.
2. Therapy with two therapists: A team of therapists held two sessions per week over a period of five to six months, 35 sessions in all.
3. Therapy with one therapist: A male or female therapist conducted sessions as above.
4. Therapy with two therapists in the group of couples: One session per week was conducted for five to six months.

   Interviews and tests to control therapy were carried out at six different times:

1. First preliminary examination. After the first examination and after indication from the Department of Sex Research at least three months but not more than twelve months before the start of therapy.
2. Second preliminary examination. Just before start of therapy after the first discussions with therapists.
3. First post-examination. Immediately after therapy.
4. Second post-examination. Three months after end of therapy.
5. Third post-examination. One year after end of therapy.
6. Fourth post-examination. Two and a half years after end of therapy.

Three areas were assessed:

1. Sexual symptoms, sexual functioning, sexual behaviour i.e. frequenty of coitus, petting, masturbation, sexual desires, sexual appetence, sexual practices, satisfaction with sexuality, and attitudes to sexuality as well as any changes in this area.
2. General relationship between the partners, i.e. understanding, affection, openness, ability to communicate, joint activities, and changes in this area.
3. General psychiatric condition i.e. psychosomatic symptoms, tendency towards depression, emotional liability, self-acceptance, etc., and changes in this area.

In all three areas data were collected by several observers using different methods such as interviews, assessment scales, questionnaires, and psychological tests.

I will not examine the results in any further detail here as they have been fully described and commented on by Arentewicz and Schmidt (1980). In general the following can be said: Provided that the therapists are experienced, therapy is to a large extent successful and the results are sufficiently stable. There were no statistical differences in effectiveness between the various treatment settings. The parallel psychodiagnostic examinations do not give grounds for variations in indication, either for individual settings or for the prognosis. Finally, apart from and independently of the resulting reduction and elimination of symptoms, couple therapy leads to the reduction of neurotic tendencies in the so-called symptom carrier and in the partner.

Psychiatric patients

Technically speaking all our patients are psychiatric patients since our research team is a Department of the Psychiatric Clinic and appointments for consultation can only be made through the psychiatric out-patients' clinic. Some patients were transferred from in-patient wards for treatment at our department as soon as out-patient treatment was considered possible. Couple therapy does not seem to be easily applicable during in-patient treatment. In practical terms, every fourth couple was involved in particularly complex circumstances at the start of therapy. That is, in addition to the sexual symptoms, patients were suffering from obvious neurological or psychosomatic illnesses, neuroses, deviant forms of behaviour, physical handicaps, and ailments following disfiguring operations. The spectrum ranges from disfigurative dwarfism with funnel chest and gibbus formation to blindness, symptoms of withdrawal from severe alcoholism or drug addiction, multiple sclerosis, neurodermatitis, ulcerous colitis together with sadomasochistic partner arrangements and sadomasochistic or fetishistic fantasies and other deviant forms of behaviour. The most frequently appearing psychiatric illnesses were phasic depression, severe obsessive–compulsive neurosis, and post-psychotic states.

The brief description of the three case histories following illustrates the types of couples treated.

Case history 1 The wife complained of severe endogenous depression with paranoid episodes. The couple has been married for ten years and both husband and wife are in their late 20s. The husband is a glazier and his wife a part-time phono-typist. They have a ten-year-old daughter. The wife has never had an orgasm either through petting or coitus and has never masturbated, saying that her body is completely devoid of feelings and that she only feels molested or bored by sexual intercourse. She might 'just as well read a newspaper'. Sometimes, she feels pain during intercourse. The patient does not know who her mother is since the latter was strictly confined to hospital owing to an endogenous psychosis. The patient was herself raped when still a child. Her only other sexual experiences have been with her husband with whom she joined up because, simply, she was happy that anyone should want to keep her company and she wanted to compensate the other's presence. She soon became pregnant and, during pregnancy, morose. She underwent psychiatric treatment for almost ten years and was an in-patient for some time. Two or three years ago, she experienced particularly acute depressive phases with paranoid episodes and has been treated for the last nine years with neuroleptic medication in high doses for depression. At the start of therapy, she had been for some months on Dapotum 3 ml every two weeks, Haldol 30 drops three times a day, Tavor 1 mg three times a day, Librium 10 mg three times a day, and Akineton 1 Tb twice a day. At the start of therapy she also lacked drive turning into apathy, had disturbed sleep, severely depressive ill-humour, a tendency to relapse into tearful decompensation, and pronounced extrapyramidal symptoms which were partly induced by the medication. The previous history of the husband showed a tendency of retarded or even no ejaculation at all. The relationship is characterized by the wife's demanding attitude towards her husband who mothers and spoils her and her lack of any self-reliance.

Case history 2 The man is dependent on alcohol and drugs. Both partners are in their early 40s, the husband a master tailor and his wife an assistant dietitian. They have been married for almost 20 years and have one child. They are quite clearly motivated to enter therapy principally for erectile dysfunction and the tendency to ejaculate prematurely from which both disorders the husband has been suffering for the last three years. The genesis and circumstances can, however, no longer be precisely determined as they have both had sexual intercourse or attempted intercourse with one another at the most two or three times a year for several years. The sexual difficulties are overshadowed by an overwhelming number of somatic and psychological symptoms and the stagnant state of their relationship. The husband has often been ill since childhood and has spent several years in hospital. He was injured in the war and still suffers from the effects. As a young man he was once involved in a violent fight between drunkards and was kicked so hard in the testicles that one of them had to be amputated, whereupon the other became somewhat atrophic. Furthermore, the patient suffers from hypertension, aches in the chest and convulsive stomach and intestinal pains. A surgical operation for the latter is already being considered. In the last few years he has lost 25 pounds in weight and has hardly slept at night. His pronounced inferiority feelings can be traced to his childhood and were aggravated to the utmost by the loss of one of his testicles. This was such a shock to his sense of identity that he became a dipsomaniac and, what is more, indiscriminately consumed every tranquillizer and analgesic he could lay his hands on. He has as a result often been under psychiatric care. His dependence on drugs led to hefty marital arguments after which he reacted with suicide threats and, once, with a spectacular suicide attempt. The wife, who on first appearance makes a far more robust impression, also has a history plagued by illness. She has pains in her joints and has had them treated for years by several doctors simultaneously, without any improvement. Moreover, her back is badly disfigured by a large lipoma and she had been on sick-leave for 15 months prior to therapy owing to serious bronchitis. They made each other's acquaintance at a spa, and both wanted to put their unhappy past experiences behind them and to marry quickly. The marriage was marred from the start by crises and illnesses, reconciliations and breakdowns. Sexuality is purely functional, its only purpose being reproduction. This function at least, with the help of hormone substitution and artificial insemination, was fulfilled. However, the child alone could not bear the burden of holding the marriage together. The problems continued to exist in the old, typical form. She is the suffering and helpful mother and wife, who sacrifices her health for husband and daughter. He is mortally ill, full of inferiority complexes, and convinced that he is of no use at all to a woman like her. He pumps himself full of medicaments and alcohol until he is delirious and in danger of suffocating in his own vomit, but is always saved just in time by his wife.

Case history 3 Owing to a sadistic perversion the husband in this relationship is in danger of killing his own wife. He is 30 years old and is a customs officer. He complains of having had occasional erectile dysfunction and retarded or no ejaculation at all ever since his first experiences with sexual intercourse. The erectile dysfunction has become so acute in the last three years that sexual intercourse is no longer possible in spite of regular attempts. He thinks his sexual dysfunction and his lack of sexual appetence and attraction have existed since his childhood. He has been masturbating regularly since he was seven years old and his impression is that retarded ejaculation did not occur then. However, to be able to masturbate he has to lie on his left side 'curled up like an embryo' in the fold of his bed, tuck his penis between his thighs and has to picture sadistic rape scenes in his mind. Every other position or manual stimulation and dispensing with fantasies all fail to arouse him. His similarly aged wife, who does not hold a job and has no sexual dysfunction, has been married to him for four years. He made her acquaintance through a matchmaking agency, looking more for a partner in life and not quite so much for sexual contact. He gradually came to enjoy petting but, if he got an erection at all, indulged in sexual intercourse with reluctance and for his wife's sake alone. Seminal emission, however, never occurs. The whole affair is extremely distressing for both of them and turns into a strenuous effort. The only way he manages to be aroused at all during sexual intercourse is by imagining that he is being brutal to his wife. He once bit and throttled her. At work he is submissive and unable to stand up for himself. When arguing with his superiors, he loses his powers of concentration and has for years been suffering from duodenal ulcers. These have been mildly treated but still recur at regular intervals. Ever since the occurrence of this malady, he has avoided attempting sexual intercourse. His opinion of the relationship, which by the way both partners agree to be good, is that he should be happy; his wife has not left him because of the sexual difficulties.

The case histories described should only be understood as examples. We admitted these and similar other couples to our treatment programme for two reasons:

1. We consider ourselves to be the psychiatric department of this hospital and feel responsible for the treatment of these patients. In extreme cases we were able to fall back on the experience and in-patient treatment in the clinic (as in case history 2).
2. We also take these patients because the intake criteria propagated by other research teams, as for example an intact relationship, are criteria that are quite likely to be chosen to increase the probability of a particularly high rate of success which, in turn, is beneficial to the therapist's prestige. However, it had not been proven that such criteria of selection are empirically justified or necessary.

Our results show that psychiatric illnesses do not necessarily represent contraindication for couple therapy. But they do require a high degree of therapeutic skill and flexibility in working with the more or less standardized methods and aims of therapy.

Our aims as regards the psychotic patient in case history 1 were directed less at the intervention on the level of 'orgasm during sexual intercourse' than at the development of pregenital sexual activities. This was intended to give the woman an opportunity to feel more protected in her relationship with her husband without having to feel afraid of losing her sense of identity. This further lessens the ever present danger of aggravating the psychosis and enables problems between the partners to be alleviated. It was possible steadily to reduce neuroleptic medication, a step which had also to be taken in order to put an end to affective suppression caused by medication. At the end of therapy the patient only took very small and in effect merely cosmetic doses in comparison to the previous eight years. The dosage level did not need to be reassessed until a follow-up examination three years later. The patient had not suffered from depression during those three years, was capable of making more and stiffer demands on herself and was livelier, having never felt a stronger sense of inner harmony. She mentioned, only in passing, the fact that she now reached orgasm regularly during intercourse feeling that this was of less importance to her than the over-all improvement in the relationship.

With his chaotic behaviour the man in case history 2, who was addicted to drugs and alcohol, continually forced the therapists to modify the therapeutic concept. At sessions he sat doubled up with physical pains, turned up in a drunken state and used every means to try and distract attention from the problems with his partner. He once came with his pockets stuffed full of tablets and threatened to take his own life. No longer wishing to stay in the clinic, he eventually had to be forcibly admitted because he was in immediate danger of committing suicide. The chaos of his barren relationship affected the therapists' mood and induced them to take new action. An improvement first set in after this situation, which was just as distressing for the therapists, had been discussed in the supervision group and after the couple had consequently agreed that the therapists would in future concentrate only on treatment of the specific sexual problem. After 34 sessions, distributed over one year, the couple were able to enjoy regular sexual intercourse to the satisfaction of both. The relationship was in general more relaxed and the husband's dependence on alcohol and drugs increasingly lost its effect.

I will now discontinue the causistic investigation of these disorders and present one or two general conclusions and suggestions.

CONCLUDING REMARKS AND SUGGESTIONS

Delineating and isolating the sexual symptom and its specific treatment within the scope of couple therapy is useful and effective

It is hardly necessary to expound further on this measure which is none the less not without its dangers. This can be most clearly seen to emerge in developments in the United States that are slowly taking hold in West Germany. Sex therapists and clinics are sprouting out of the ground like mushrooms and sex weekends and workshops are being turned into an aphrodisiac for run-down relationships. The sex therapists organize their skills into a leisure industry of human enhancement and marital enrichment programmes, and lend it the stamp of scientific legitimacy with academic titles such as 'Dr. med. sex'. Perfecting sexual performance, whether by following the concept of Wilhelm Reich or Herbert Marcuse, is the quickest way to batter the last remnants of sexual pleasure to death. Anyone who is involved in the therapeutic treatment of sexual dysfunctions is always in danger of being sucked in by tendencies such as these. The best method of resisting this temptation is by actively avoiding over-specialization and turning away from the main concept of 'sexual growth programmes' and instead turning towards the treatment of more complicated disorders.

Excluding psychiatric patients from couple therapy is unprofitable and unfounded

It may have been useful previously to delineate the object of research when scientifically testing a method. And it was perhaps once advantageous to produce 'cosmetically' first class statistics showing successful results. But the moment for therapists and patients to start working against the atomization of their spheres of experience has long been passed. Masters and Johnson can be credited for having disproved Freud's thesis that every symptom was merely the tip of an iceberg. However, there is little use in throwing the baby out with the bathwater. Sexual dysfunctions frequently appear in conjunction with other complaints or pathological symptoms. Our impression is that this is often the case with psychiatric patients, a fact to which psychiatrists had until recently turned a blind eye. If one considers that the integrity of many psychiatric patients' personalities is constantly endangered by psychotic collapse, that every shift in the proximity-distance equilibrium shakes the entire foundations of their psychic condition, it is hardly surprising that psychiatric patients also have sexual problems. Moreover, sexual relationships set high demands on partners to withstand the extreme fluctuations between merging and separating.

If couple therapy is understood as one form of psychotherapy among others and not merely as sexual plumbing, there is no reason why it should be denied psychiatric patients, irrespective of any pseudo-scientific arguments. Psychiatric illnesses do not invalidate indication for couple therapy.

Psychiatric illness in conjunction with sexual difficulties is sufficient ground for indication for couple therapy, if the patient and his or her partner consent

Before expounding on this thesis I am obliged to guard against a likely misunderstanding. I am not interested in opening up a new market for sex therapy, nor in embarking on specialist areas such as sex and couple therapy for the blind and the emotionally disturbed or physically handicapped, and so on. Quite the contrary; our experiences have demonstrated that treatment brings about a statistically significant lessening of neurotic and psychophysiological secondary symptoms in general psychic stabilization. This is even the case when the dysfunction could not be eliminated or only partially so. In this sense couple therapy has a partly specific, partly unspecific effect which can be judged to be positive. This indeterminate effect can be turned to good account in post-ward treatment and for prophylactic treatment of relapses in psychiatric patients.

Considering the catastrophic situation of in-patients and out-patients in psychiatric care, even a high unspecific effect amounts to a considerable gain. Furthermore, it is rewarding for the therapist to see a patient, whose emotional life had previously been tied down with chemicals, laughing freely and spontaneously and feeling innervated by the relationship with his or her partner. The selection of patients is not only a question of scientific accuracy but also a political question.

REFERENCES

Arentewicz, G., and Schmidt, G. (eds.) (1980) *Sexuell Gestörte Beziehungen. Konzept und Technik der Paratherapie.* Springer, Berlin, Heidelberg, New York.

LoPicollo, J., and Lobitz, W. C. (1973) Behaviour therapy of sexual dysfunctions, in Hammerlynck, L. A., Handy, L. C., and Mash, I. J. (eds.) *Behavioral Chance: Methodology, Concept, and Practice*, Research Press, Champaign, Illinois, pp. 349–358.
Masters, W. H., and Johnson, V. E. (1970) *Human Sexual Inadequacy* Little, Brown, Boston.

V. LEARNING THEORY AND MANAGEMENT OF CHILDREN'S DISORDERS

Learning Theory Approaches to Psychiatry
Edited by John Boulougouris
© 1982 John Wiley & Sons Ltd

18. BEHAVIOUR MODIFICATION OF HYPERACTIVE CHILDREN WITH CONDUCT DISORDERS: THE USE OF TRIADIC MODEL INTERVENTIONS IN HOME-SETTINGS

Martin Herbert

It is very difficult to select what to say in a relatively brief chapter about six or seven years' work with children in their natural environments—mainly 'own home' or residential care settings, and less often, in classroom situations. Natural environment interventions, in contrast to clinic-based treatment, seek to utilize the on-going and intensive influence of those in closest everyday contact with the client in attempting to modify deviant behaviour and teach new skills and behavioural repertoires (O'Dell, 1974). The triadic model, as it is called, by-passes the problem of generalizing improvements from the consulting room to the outside world. Parents and teachers—as primary mediators of change—are *in situ* most of the time, and are in a position to apply contingencies in a variety of situations. Whatever the apparent theoretical advantages of the triadic model, there are many practical difficulties associated with its application. So I hope I will be excused for emphasizing the practical difficulties of working with populations of $n > 1$, and in natural settings.

Natural setting work means, in effect, 'unnatural' experimental investigations, as it is so difficult to specify and control pre- and post-treatment conditions with precision. However, as Repucci and Saunders (1974) so forcibly argue, the boundaries of behaviour modification are expanding, and the crucial issues to be resolved include the social application of behavioural methods. They make the point that in the natural environment the behaviour therapist (modifier) encounters a wide range of problems that do not relate directly to theoretical issues in behaviour modification and which are absent or minimal in the laboratory or clinical research situation.

This chapter presents a few comments on the feasibility aspect of our work at the Child Treatment Research Unit (C.T.R.U.), based at the University of Leicester. Further details of the approach and its efficacy are published elsewhere. (C.T.R.U. Research Reports 1–7*; Herbert, 1978, 1981; Herbert and Iwaniec, 1981).

I can best underline the validity of Repucci and Saunders' caveat about the triadic model by instancing the scepticism of many people I meet in various helping professions who have tried (to take one example) to treat nocturnal enuresis with behavioural methods—i.e. with the bell-and-pad conditioning technique. Their experience, contrary to ours in residential settings (where we have achieved 90% success rates) and in own-home settings (88.2% success rates), and to the findings of many research-based investigations, is disappointing. On enquiry, it often turns out that parents have been handed a bell-and-pad and a leaflet of instructions and told to get on with it. Small wonder this well-tested method fails in the absence of careful assessment, monitoring, and follow-up. Many things can go wrong with even this allegedly 'simple' technique. A great deal of attention must be given to practical details (Herbert, 1981) and remedial, or better still pre-emptive, action taken by careful monitoring and follow-up—when things go wrong as they so often do in the 'unruly' setting of home or classroom. There, one has limited control over contingencies of reinforcement, not to mention the vicissitudes of day-to-day living.

However, I do not wish to dwell on practical difficulties associated with these or other problems such as encopresis, phobias, and 'failure to thrive' with which we have been concerned at the C.T.R.U. Our work with hyperactive conduct disordered children—a notoriously infractory group—provides apt examples of the advantages and disadvantages of working with caregivers as the main mediators of change. Our earliest data (measures of change and debriefing sessions with individuals and members of a parents' group) were generated by an evolving programme carried out on 117 families (79 boys, 38 girls; median age: five years; age range 18 months to 16 years). Problems included aggression, extreme non-compliance, destructiveness, disruptiveness, delinquent acts, and a wide variety of high rate, high intensity behaviours. (A wide range of behaviours are referred to as conduct problems and include moderately troublesome acts as well as severe antisocial behaviours ('conduct disorder'). Most of the children in this sample (83%) manifested problem behaviour beyond the realm of 'merely bothersome' and were causing serious disruption within the family. In many cases they were perceived by their parents to be 'out of control'.

It should be said that the C.T.R.U. was set up as a service-orientated agency devoted to the training of social work and clinical psychology students in behaviour modification, and to research into the feasibility and efficacy of triadic model work with various childhood problems (Herbert, 1978). The unit was staffed by graduate students under the supervision of a clinical psychologist/behaviour therapist (the author). These students occupied the counsellor or consultant role (Tharp and Wetzel, 1969).

Broadly speaking our studies of this large sample and a group based on a smaller sample of referrals (n = 36) using a more rigorous evaluative methodology (Herbert et al., 1982) have produced similar results: approximately 60% improved satisfactorily (as rated by parents, therapists, independent assessor, and on graphical records); 20% showed moderate improvement; 20% displayed no change.

It is difficult to provide a base rate for conduct problems because of difficulties of definition and a paucity of longitudinal evidence. But unlike the development of fears and many other problems of childhood, there is not the same tendency for the conduct problems to be transitory. Writers such as Robins (1966) suggest that by ages seven or eight years the child with extreme antisocial aggressive patterns of behaviour is at quite considerable risk of continuing on into adolescence and indeed adulthood with serious deviancy of one kind or another.

Unfortunately, there is insufficient space to explain how the unit began to see large numbers of children under that age (some above) who seemed to be on that slippery slope toward manifesting serious problem behaviour. Of course, I have no way of knowing what would have happened to these children without treatment. The common complaint of the parents was that they had had trouble with their offspring from early on in life. They had been mollified at first by the experts' predictions: 'Don't worry he'll grow out of it ... Just do this ... or that ...' (prescriptions couched in vague and global terminology). Instead the problems seemed to get worse as the child grew stronger and more mobile. Parents looked forward to school-going or the child's teens with foreboding as their 'delinquencies' would be labelled and the finger pointed unerringly at the 'bad homes' they had allegedly provided. (In fact, not a few of these homes were good or well-meaning.)

Some of these youngsters had already been labelled hyperactive. (I would prefer not to get into that vexed semantic question except that we developed a scale in order to reduce some of the subjectivity associated with the label.) The problems complained of were a mixture of high rate, high intensity coercive behaviours which were compellingly attention-demanding and disruptive. The addition of extreme non-compliance made for unhappy parent–child interactions and a fraught family atmosphere, including (in not a few cases) deteriorating marital relationships and growing social isolation. It was not long before what seemed to me the 'compelling logic' of looking at these children and their despairing parents on their own territory forced me out of the hospital and the unit at the university and into their homes. It was also at the request of the more articulate parents. 'I wish the doctor could see how really bad he is at home or at the supermarket ... I'm sure he doesn't believe me ... thinks I'm a neurotic mother. I don't think my husband does sometimes. He comes back when Johnny's tired out and sees the best of him.'

At this point I would like to digress for a moment to reflect briefly on child development and the process of learning to become a social being. One of the most pleasant ways of reflecting about the socialization (and indeed, behaviour modification) of children is to lie on the beach, half asleep, surrounded by parents and their children. There are so many opportunities for disruptive (not to mention deviant) actions on the part of the innovative youngster. There is sand to throw in the face of his brothers and sisters, buckets and spades to fight over, ice-creams to pester for. There is the possibility of burying his sleeping father alive. Then there are the exciting adventures which bring potential danger: floating the rubber boat out to sea, wandering away and getting lost. There are so many rules to learn and obey!

Lying there and listening drowsily to mothers (and fathers) at their work as child-rearers, care-givers, trainers, one is impressed by the enormous input, the seemingly endless 'lessons' whereby parents remind, instruct, and modify their offsprings' actions. (It makes one's once- or twice-a-week input on the dyadic model seem puny and somewhat presumptuous.) But the main point I wish to make with the image of the seaside, is the way that it highlights the pleasure (and frustrations) of work on the triadic model.

The pleasure lies in the fact that parents are very familiar with the essentials of behaviour modification; in fact the behaviour therapist is likely to suffer from the 'Ooh, I've tried that!' rejoinder every time he suggests a change strategy. After all parents are applied learning theorists in an informal (and sometimes uninformed) manner. They reward and punish, instruct, model behaviour, give reasons, and explanations (i.e. use inductive methods) in order to change, instruct, and generally rear their offspring so as to be social beings. When the behavioural approach is explained to parents and teachers in an uncondescending but straightforward manner, it seems to have face validity for them. It removes the demystification and obfuscation which are features of so many therapies—and this is crucial if they are going to adopt their rightful role as the significant mediators and maintainers of change. After all, learning occurs within a social context; rewards, punishments, and other events are mediated by human agents and within attachment systems, and are not simply the impersonal consequences of behaviour. Unfortunately—and it is the case with all forms of learning—the very processes which help the child adapt to life can, under certain circumstances, contribute to his maladjustment. An immature child who learns by imitating an adult is not necessarily to know when it is deviant behaviour that is being modelled. His mother may unwittingly reinforce his tantrums by paying attention to them.

If it is accepted that many deviant behaviours of childhood and adulthood are acquired as a function of faulty learning processes, then there is a case for arguing that problems can most effectively be modified (and indeed, prevented) when and where they occur, by changing the 'social lessons' he receives and the reinforcing contingencies supplied by social agents. A corollary of such a proposition—especially with regard to the conduct disorders which involve a profound inability (or unwillingness) to comply with rules—is to treat the child within, and through, the family (the main agents of socialization) rather than removing him from the setting in which the problems occur.

Returning to the seaside: it is obvious that parents' behaviour training 'programmes' are not designed on the same premises as behaviour therapists' formal programmes. The effectiveness of the latter are measured by the maintenance of improvements over long periods of time. Clearly parents (or most of them) and, perhaps even behaviour therapists in their role as parents, do not harbour the illusion that child-training is made up of one-off programmatic efforts which have failed when the child reverts to the old, or discovers new, misdemeanours. And perhaps it is here—in notions of 'cure'—that the ubiquitous medical model has slipped back into the consciousness of behaviour modifiers. It has some, but only limited relevance in the emotional and behavioural problems of childhood (Herbert, 1974). The fact is that parents (and teachers) resign themselves with varying degrees of fatalism to repeating the lessons of socialization. They recognize that time-scales vary, depending on the age and maturity of the child and the nature of the behavioural skill or task; parents should not (and usually do not) expect the child to acquire and maintain certain lessons without setbacks and repetitions.

Meditating on the beach about the initiating activities of the infants in the near vicinity, reminds one of a child-training issue of note. The child's response to his world is much more then a simple reaction to his environment. He is actively engaged in attempts to organize and structure his world. Any truly transactional model (Herbert, 1980) must stress the changing character of the environment and of the organism as an active participant in its own development. Interpretations of socialization in terms of social reinforcement have shared (in the past) a common view of the infant as an essentially passive organism whose character is moulded solely by the impact of environment upon genetic predispositions. This vertical model presupposes a child who is part of a one-way traffic in which he is under the control of a socializing agent who dispenses rewards and punishments (Zigler and Child, 1969). There is evidence (Harper, 1975)—and the therapist cannot afford to forget it—that the direction of effects of socialization is not always downward, from parent to child. Parents are not the sole possessors of power and influence within the family. What is obvious from recent studies is that important individual differences are manifested in early infancy, among them being temperamental attributes.

It is the author's strong, but still tentative, conviction that a significant factor in the development of some conduct problems is a temperamental or congenital factor (and in particular one to do with activity) which has powerfully modified the parents' expectations and the manner in which they have reared a remarkably demanding infant. Early learning is shaped in such a way that the range of coercive tactics (crying, screaming, wilful tantrums, non-compliance) which are common to all young children are not relinquished in this kind of child as he grows older—because of the way in which his potent behaviour has been mismanaged (Herbert, 1978).

Most parents, with little or no training—and I believe parenting to be in large part a skill—rear their children into broadly pro-social, norm-abiding adults (with the help of other socializing agents). There seems to be a fair amount of latitude in learning conditions for the child with an intact central nervous system, body, and a relatively unvolcanic temperament. For them, parental inconsistency, double-binds, unclear rules, etc. seem no more than a minor hindrance in the business of growing up. For others, predisposed to problem formation by handicaps, temperamental lability, or learning deficits, a more predictable and persistent learning environment becomes essential. The demand characteristics of such children—the high rate, high-intensity behaviours of a coercive kind so often associated with handicap—sadly (and too often) shape up an environment which is fraught, unpredictable, and unpersevering!

Empirical findings suggest an interesting hypothesis (see Patterson, 1975): that there is a curvilinear relationship between activity level of the child and the acquisition of socially acceptable behaviour. Up to moderately high levels of activity, the child's behaviour will call forth an increasing number of reactions from peers and adults. Assuming that these reactions are, by and large, positive, this probably means that the active ordinary child will acquire social skills at a faster rate than the less active child. It is further assumed that extremely high rates of behaviour are aversive for other people; thus the reactions from society are more likely to be punitive.

In this situation, the child functioning at very high levels of activity is quite likely to be punished even when he is displaying socially acceptable behaviour, e.g. friendliness or co-operation. This higher ratio of punishment to reinforced behaviour for the hyperactive child may well result in his acquiring social behaviour at a slow pace (Patterson, 1975). According to Cruickshank (1968) the basic need of hyperactive children is for success—success is something in which adults and adult society genuinely believe. This we try to build into our treatment programmes.

I mentioned earlier the frustrations of doing home-based behaviour modification: notably the 'I've tried it' syndrome. This is the price of using concepts and methods that are on a continuum with their day-to-day child training practices: 'Time-out?' 'Oooh, I've tried that'; 'Response-cost?' 'I've tried that'; 'Over-correction?' 'That didn't work', and so on. Of course, parents may not be aware of the small print of learning principles: matters of timing, the need for careful specification, and contingency analysis.

This chapter is intended to cover 'Behaviour modification in the natural home setting'. I can imagine many of the parents of the parents' group that we were later to form, laughing derisively at that term: 'natural' home. Many felt that theirs were highly unnatural homes and that family life had become a travesty: rows, social isolation, a sense of being trapped, depression, feelings of being ineffectual failures as parents. Most frightening were the fears and fantasies of some parents of doing something extremely violent to the child.

We have found almost invariably that parents welcome our use of their homes as the base for working with them and training them. Gardner (1976) describes various levels of training. He considered the generalist level (the generalist has the 'know-how' to apply theory and techniques to a wide spectrum of problems with a minimum of supervision) to be the most common level for training parents. It may be a desideratum for parents dealing with multiple and fairly persistent or chronic childhood problems (e.g. conduct disordered, mentally subnormal, or autistic children).

The rationale of our desire (not always fulfilled in practice) to train parents to the generalist level was the belief that the parents' on-going contact with the child and possession of new skills might facilitate generalization of treatment effects across time. (We are researching into the cost-effectiveness and cost-benefits of training parents in different ways.) Sadly, the evidence in the area of temporal generalization is mixed: positive with regard to long-term persistence of favourable effects in some

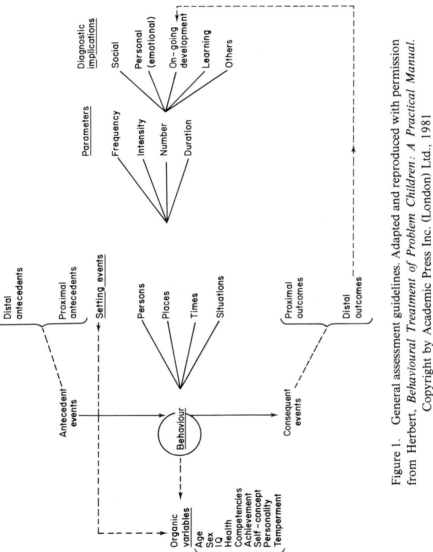

Figure 1. General assessment guidelines. Adapted and reproduced with permission from Herbert, *Behavioural Treatment of Problem Children: A Practical Manual.* Copyright by Academic Press Inc. (London) Ltd., 1981

studies (Donofrio, 1976; Rinn *et al.*, 1975), negative or minimal in others (Ferber *et al.*, 1974; Johnson and Christensen, 1975). A further hope is that thorough parent-training will enhance the transfer of skills applied to one problem in the child's behavioural repertoire area to novel problems manifested by the same child. This expectation (Patterson *et al.*, 1973) is difficult to translate into reality. The evidence is a little more positive when it comes to generalization across children (Patterson *et al.*, 1972; Resick *et al.*, 1976).

A conceptual framework for our work with families (Herbert, 1981) is summarized in Figure 1. It is essentially a social learning approach to assessment and treatment. Here is the kind of information we will be seeking with the family's help.

During the initial interview with the child and both parents (a crucial therapeutic configuration we have found in families where there are two parents), we explain who we are and how we work. It is C.T.R.U. policy to raise some of the major issues generated by a triadic behavioural approach: the concept of a genuine therapeutic partnership; our desire to share our knowledge and thinking with the parents, to take into account their own expertise based on longstanding knowledge of the child, and also to communicate the commitment we have to look at the ethical implications of any plans to institute changes within the family. This requires a role of advocacy on behalf of the child, and requires a good understanding of developmental norms and the social and psychological implications of behaviour change. If the idea of sharing information and knowledge is not to be mere cant and lipservice, then it requires a genuine democratic participation by the family in goal-setting and discussion of the feasibility (and ethical implications) of using specific behavioural techniques. We invite parents to the case conference. There is a technical pay-off in sharing information; a reduction in the number of drop-outs from treatment (Baekeland and Lundwall, 1975). There may, however, be crucial variables in the style of training (e.g. didactic versus a participant approach) which influence drop-out rates. Parental drop-out from training research reviewed by O'Dell (1975) suggests that it can be as high as 70%. At the C.T.R.U. drop-out numbers have proved negligible.

In all there are 20 assessment and treatment steps (Herbert, 1981). Table 1 shows the first six steps concerned with the preliminary screening.

In furtherance of our philosophy of sharing knowledge (and, indeed, our uncertainties where they exist), the 'commonsense' and familiar aspects of child management are stressed. It is emphasized that if a behavioural treatment is felt to be appropriate then this is likely to involve altering the consequences of the child's

Table 1.   Preliminary screening

Step 1	Explain yourself and how you work
Step 2	Identify the problems
Step 3a	Construct a problem profile
Step 3b	Define and refine specific target behaviours
Step 4	Discover the desired outcomes
Step 5	Identify the child's assets
Step 6	Establish problem priorities

problem behaviour. But it is also stressed that the parents should be prepared not only to change their present responses to the child's supposedly maladaptive behaviours, but also to initiate new behaviours provided that they are not required to do anything distasteful or contrary to their values as parents.

It is demonstrated how problems are not encapsulated within the child but are contingent upon things he has learned within a social context, including their own actions and reactions to him. Many parents seem to perceive their children as active volcanoes, erupting at odd times (and far too frequently) with bad behaviour. We warn parents that we will require them to do a good deal of 'homework'; monitoring the child's (and their own) behaviours along lines that we will teach them. Their initial dismay is usually (we have learnt) replaced by a sense of pleasure and 're-moralization' at being actively engaged in the assessment (and later) the treatment of their child. Some report that the act of recording tense situations provides a cooling-off interlude, time to think. One problem for the experimentalist is that it is difficult to hold some parents to a baseline period. They 'get the idea' and wish to initiate their new-found understanding in practical child-management strategies. But this is hardly surprising. After all we underline the point that we are not there as 'experts' to take over the burden of the child's problem from the parents but that it is a co-operative venture with a major part of the responsibility rightfully in their hands.

Parents are cautioned that there could be disagreement over treatment objectives (reservations on the part of the C.T.R.U. in the negotiations about what behaviour to modify) and finally, that despite a prolonged assessment procedure there could be no guarantee (at the conclusion of the assessment) that a behavioural treatment programme would even be considered appropriate.

But we have jumped ahead. At the point that the parents agree that they can accept the conditions attached to the C.T.R.U. intervention (e.g. keeping records, keeping to agreed plans, etc.) the team goes ahead with a full behavioural assessment and analysis. The rationale for collecting this data is provided. A brief account is given (with down-to-earth examples) of the theoretical model used by the agency, pointing out how problem behaviour, like normal behaviour, can be acquired through failures or anomalies of learning and how such problems might be alleviated by practical strategies based on theories of learning and development. Table 2 contains Steps 7 to 15 which are worked through with the parents and child—the baseline phase.

Parents frequently tell us at the debriefing interviews that this information and the 'insights' they gain from a more rigorous definition (and monitoring) of antisocial and prosocial behaviour, mark the beginning of change in their interactions with their child and (for some) a growing sense of competence. Despite our best intentions the baseline period is seldom therapeutically inert. About 10% show reductions in target behaviours during the baseline period and maintain the improvement, at least over the four weeks we keep in touch with them.

In initiating baseline work our preliminary task is to specify precisely what the allegedly maladaptive behaviours are, defining them in terms of their frequency, intensity, number and duration, and the meaning (or sense†) they have for the child

Table 2.   Baseline phase

Step 7	Specify situations
Step 8	Assess the extent and severity of the problem
Step 9	Provide client with appropriate recording material
Step 10a	Find out more about the behaviour
Step 10b	Find out how intense the behaviour is
Step 10c	How many problems are being manifested by the Child?
Step 10d	Find out about the duration of the problem
Step 10e	What sense or meaning is there in the problem behaviour?
Step 11	Assess the contingencies
Step 12	Identify reinforcers
Step 13	Assess organismic variables
Step 14a	Arrive at a diagnostic decision
Step 14b	Formulate objectives
Step 14c	Draw up a verbal agreement or written contract
Step 15	Formulate clinical hypotheses

(FINDS). (Figure 1) The analysis is very much (but not exclusively) focused on what is called the 'ABC' sequence. An analysis is made (by ourselves and the parents) of environmental conditions (and physical factors) leading up to, and immediately preceding the occurrence of the problem behaviour, and those that follow the performance of such behaviour. In this way we try to discover the antecedent stimuli (A) and consequences (C) which serve as eliciting or discriminative stimuli and thus trigger and maintain problem behaviour (B) in terms of learning and behavioural principles which will be understandable to the family.

During the early assessment period the key word is 'what'. (Herbert, 1981). The parent is taught to think sequentially and in terms of interacting systems. What is the child doing? What are other persons doing? Under what conditions in the family are these behaviours (or interactions) emitted? Parents tend to press for quick prescriptions, and answers (which it is important to resist) to the fascinating questions 'how?' and 'why?'. Explanations of the need for painstaking data collection prior to formulating hypotheses are usually accepted.

One of the problems in triadic work concerns the reliability of parental (and in the case of self-monitoring) child observations. We attempt to check on these recordings during our home visits so as to enhance the confidence we place in the data base. We find it helps to write down the behaviour to be recorded (with symbols and definitions) on large sheets of paper on the kitchen wall—as reminders to the parents and/or child. The assessment of these events is directed towards the precise identification of the antecedent, outcome, and symbolic conditions which control the problem behaviour.

At all times the parent is encouraged to give descriptive examples (preferably recent ones) of the problems and confrontations in specific and observable terms; she is reminded to avoid inferential language such as 'he's aggressive' or 'she tries to get me down'. A technique used to tease out family interactions and target behaviours is the 'typical day' in the life of the child and the family. It is worked through in minute detail, pinpointing those areas which provided the times and places at which, and the persons with whom, they occurred. We are at pains to find out (as diplomatically as possible) whether there is someone, say a granny, with whom the child does not display his deviant behaviour. This is good news as the child is capable of self-control and we may be able to learn from that situation.

Parents tend to express their concern about their child's shortcomings as statements about problems and/or desired outcomes. Such initial comments about desired outcomes provide the raw material for the formulation (later) of more specific goals and objectives. We make a note of who is complaining about particular problems, who desires a given outcome, the level of agreement/disagreement between parents and child with regard to how they would like things to be different, and the implications of change in the direction of the desired outcome. (Who benefits? Does anyone lose?).

The literature on behaviour modification—as it applies to children's conduct disorders—reflects a relative neglect of antecedent events. In their preoccupation with consequences of behaviour and, hence, operant procedures, behaviour modifiers sometimes overlook environmental controlling stimuli and the possibilities of ameliorating and restructuring the child's environment. It is helpful to observe what behaviours the parents model (consciously or unconsciously) for the child to imitate, or the confusing or weak verbal signals they give. There are other factors to be taken into account, but insufficient space here to elaborate.

Parents are usually invited to the case conference which occurs after some two or more weeks of baseline work so as to debate and finalize the plan of treatment, and to draw up a contract. Once the case conference has arrived at a formulation of the problem a detailed plan is made with the parents for the intervention, which they initiate. It is vital to warn them, if one is not to lose them, that the child is likely to get worse before he gets better—the post-extinction burst. The 'machiavellian' child is expert at producing target behaviour criterion confusion or slippage. A fairly intensive input at the beginning of a programme (providing prompts, cues, moral support, modelling, etc.) has proved invaluable in facilitating the work. We work basically with a family system: the child is viewed as part of a complex network of

Table 3.   Intervention and termination

Step 16a	Plan your treatment programme
Step 16b	Take into account non-specific therapeutic factors
Step 16c	Assess the resources for treatment
Step 17	Work out the practicalities of the treatment programme
Step 18	Evaluate the programme
Step 19	Initiate the programme
Step 20	Phase out and terminate treatment

interacting social systems any aspect of which may have a bearing on his present troubles. Thus in attempting to reach some kind of assessment and plan a programme of treatment the unit of attention is broadly conceived ($n > 1$).

Table 3 describes Steps 16 to 20 which concern the intervention and its eventual termination.

There is no set treatment formula; there is a wide choice of methods but their implementation and back-up require sensitivity, ingenuity, and creative clinical skills.

REINFORCEMENT PROGRAMME

The positive reinforcement of prosocial actions and removal of reinforcement or application of punishment contingent upon antisocial behaviours are particularly useful. Time-out from positive reinforcement (periods of five minutes for children below the age of ten years), response-cost and over-correction procedures have proved to be among the most effective sanctions (Herbert, 1978). Incentive systems (token economies) were negotiated between parents and children, and some were linked to behaviour at school. In the case of the older children (and, for some parents) we use *self-control training* (including relaxation training, desensitization of anger, role-play, behaviour rehearsal) and social-skills training. Techniques which have proved to be invaluable (Herbert, 1978) with hyperactive, impulsive children are *modelling* and *self-instruction training*—the development of children's skills in guiding their own performance by the use of self-suggestion, comments, praise, and other directives. Frequent use is made of *alternative response training*, a method that provides children with alternate modes of response to cope with provocative and disturbing situations.

Details of our results using such methods are published elsewhere (Herbert, 1978; Herbert *et al.*, 1982). To the extent that we are successful in the short-term, it is difficult to disentangle the therapeutic ingredients. This has been an evolving programme using simple AB or ABC intrasubject research designs, one in which we have learnt (and, hopefully are still learning) by our mistakes. There are many components: expectancy effects, the behavioural work itself, developmental counselling, and the growing sense of self-confidence (efficacy) that parents report as a result of their involvement in the therapy. We attend to practical matters such as arranging for baby-sitters and child-minders; we organize a playgroup and parents' group to give exhausted parents 'a break', important if they are going to have the stamina for a programme.

We are left with several problems. The main one is the technical difficulty of maintaining effects over time. Our 'failure rate' here over a year's follow-up is about one in five. All who gave us the opportunity to carry out booster programmes returned to termination levels or better. We are evaluating the role of the parents' group (with its social, experiential, and didactic functions) in facilitating temporal generalization. It certainly is a help in 'softening the blow' in the case of our failures.

Another issue we learned the hard way is the importance of reinforcing the reinforcers. We build in treats and mutual encouragement for the parents when they fulfil their tasks. It is crucial to involve the father for his practical and moral support of the mother and to allow her 'time-out' from the children. Where we did not do this we found that in one way or another the programme was subverted.

Not infrequently we have had to work at several levels, providing practical social support or advice, giving marital counselling, carrying out an individualized programme for a depressed or anxious mother. Imaginative consideration of the meaning of the programme for siblings is essential. Some have become difficult. We explain the programme to them and sometimes involve them in the payoffs. Criterion slippage is the great danger as tired mothers adopt the line of least resistance with a child and put him back on an intermittently reinforced schedule for deviant behaviour.

Fading out a programme requires careful planning although some parents pre-empt this phase and begin it 'off their own bat'. It is vital to have selected areas of change which are functional for the child. If the behaviours chosen have no natural reinforcing value for the child, and thus have no adaptive and survival functions, we are wasting everybody's time. It is our common experience that successful results have effects that ripple out well beyond the target interactions in a way that makes for happier family life.

The use of behaviour modification with hyperactive and conduct disordered children is, at very least, encouraging. In conclusion, I should like to emphasize the necessity of applying behavioural principles in a manner that is informed by developmental knowledge and theory. For example, there is substantial agreement about conditions conducive to the acquisition of standards of morality—a crucial consideration in the conduct disorders. They include firm moral demands made by parents upon their youngsters; the consistent use of sanctions; techniques of punishment that are psychological rather than physical (i.e. methods which signify or threaten withdrawal of approval and love) and an intensive use of reasoning and explanations. An understanding of factors like these should add to the efficacy of the therapist's work (Aronfreed, 1968).

NOTES

* The Child Treatment Research Unit references signify a series of unpublished reports, which are available from Professor M. Herbert, Psychology Department, University of Leicester, University Road, Leicester, LE1 7RH.

† This item concerns the perception the child has of his behaviour; the sort of 'stories' he tells himself about their antecedents and outcomes (e.g. expectancies–perceptions of payoffs).

REFERENCES

Aronfreed, J. (1968) *Conduct and Conscience*, Academic Press, New York.
Baekeland, F., and Lundwall, L. (1975) Dropping out of treatment: a critical review. *Psychological Bulletin*, **82**, 738–783.

Cruickshank, W. M. (1968) Educational implications of psychopathology in brain injured children, in Loring, J. (ed.) *Assessment of the Cerebral Palsied Child for Education*, W. Heinemann, New York, pp. 50–63.

Donofrio, A. F. (1976) Parent education vs. child psychotherapy. *Psychology in the Schools*, **13**, 176–180.

Ferber, H., Keeley, S. M., and Shemberg, K. M. (1974) Training parents in behaviour modification: outcome of problems encountered in a programme after Patterson's work *Behaviour Therapy*, **5**, 415–419.

Gardner, J. M. (1976) Training parents as behaviour modifiers, in Yen, S., and McIntire, R. (eds.), *Teaching Behaviour Modification*, Behaviordelia, Kalamazoo, Michigan.

Harper, L. V. (1975) The scope of offspring effects: from caregiver to culture. *Psychological Bulletin*, **82**, 784–801.

Herbert, M. (1974) *Emotional Problems of Development in Children*, Academic Press, London.

Herbert, M. (1978) *Conduct Disorders of Childhood and Adolescence: A Behavioural Approach to Assessment and Treatment*, John Wiley, Chichester.

Herbert, M. (1981) *Behavioural Treatment of Problem Children: A Practice Manual*, Academic Press, London; Grune & Stratton, New York.

Herbert, M. (1980) Socialization for problem resistance, in Feldman, R., and Orford, J. (eds.) *Psychological Problems: The Social Context*, John Wiley, Chichester.

Herbert, M., Holmes, A., Jehu, D., and Turner, K. (1981) *Behaviour Modification in Natural Environments*. Behaviour Research and Therapmonographs (in press).

Herbert, M., and Iwaniec, D. (1981) Behavioural psychotherapy in natural homesettings: an empirical study applied to conduct disordered and incontinent children. *Behavioural Psychotherapy*, **9**, 55–76.

Johnson, S. M., and Christensen, A. (1975) Multiple criteria follow-up of behaviour modification with families. *Abnormal Child Psychology*, **3**, 135–154.

O'Dell, S. (1974) Training parents in behaviour modification: a review *Psychological Bulletin*, **81**, 418–433.

Patterson, G. R. (1975) The coercive child: architect or victim of a coercive system?, in Hamerlynck, L., Handy, L. C., and E. J. Mash (eds.) *Behaviour Modification and Families* I. *Theory and Research*: II. *Applications and Developments*, Brunner/Mazel, New York.

Patterson, G. R., Cobb, J. A., and Ray, R. S. (1972) Direct intervention in the classroom: a set of procedures for the aggressive child, in Clark, F., Evans, D., and Hamerlynck, L. (eds.) *Implementing Behavioural Programs for Schools and Clinics*, Research Press, Champaign, Illinois, pp. 151–201.

Patterson, G. R., Cobb, J. A., and Ray, R. S. (1973) A social engineering technology for retraining the families of aggressive boys, in Adams, H. E., and Unikel, I. P. (eds.) *Issues & Trends in Behaviour Therapy*, Part II, Charles C. Thomas, Springfield, Illinois, pp. 139–210.

Repucci, N. D., and Saunders, J. T. (1974) Social psychology of behavior modification: problems of implementation in natural settings. *American Psychologist*, **29**, 649–660.

Resick, P. A., Forehand, R., and McWhorter, A. Q. (1976) The effect of parental treatment with one child on an untreated sibling. *Behaviour Therapy*, **7**, 544–548.

Rinn, R. C., Vernon, J. C., and Wise, M. J. (1975) Training parents of behaviourally-disordered children in groups: a three years' program evaluation, in Franks, C. M. (ed.) *Behavior Therapy*, Academic Press, New York, London, Vol. 6, No. 3 pp. 378–387.

Robins, L. N. (1966) *Deviant Children Grown Up*, Williams and Wilkins, Baltimore.

Tharp, R. G., and Wetzel, R. J. (1969) *Behaviour Modification in the Natural Environment*, Academic Press, London.

Zigler, E., and Child, I. L. (1969) Socialization, in Lindzey, G., and Aronson, E. (eds.) *Handbook of Social Psychology*, 2nd Edn, Addison-Wesley, Reading, Mass., Vol. 3, pp. 450–589.

Learning Theory Approaches to Psychiatry
Edited by John Boulougouris
© 1982 John Wiley & Sons Ltd

19. REDUCTION OF MEDICAL FEARS: AN INFORMATION PROCESSING ANALYSIS

Barbara Melamed

The intention of this chapter is to review research derived from our studies of modelling preparation of children for dental treatment and hospitalization for surgery in order to point out neglected areas of research. Although a multitude of studies have appeared in the literature which purport the effectiveness of advanced preparation in reducing anxiety, not many have assessed whether or not the information conveyed in this way had actually been acquired by the patients.

RATIONALE FOR PSYCHOLOGICAL PREPARATION

The need for psychological preparation of children undergoing medical or dental treatment is based on the belief that these are stressful experiences which can lead to transient or long-term psychological disturbances. The research available suggests that prepared patients are more co-operative with the health care professional if they understand what is going to happen and how they need to behave. Therefore, it is not surprising that psychological preparation has become commonplace in hospitals where children receive surgery (Peterson and Ridley-Johnson, 1980). Unfortunately, the research which exists has not evaluated important factors such as the age of the child, the effects of previous experience, or prehospital adjustment. Melamed and her colleagues (Melamed *et al.*, 1976; Melamed and Siegel, 1975; 1980) have presented data which questions the universal assumption that some form of preparation is of value for all children. They found that children under the age of seven and children with previous experience with surgery did not benefit from viewing a peer modelling film in advance of their hospitalization. There are many methodological shortcomings in addition to those already mentioned. The instruments to measure the children's anxiety vary considerably in validity and reliability. The use of retrospective parent reports and global ratings of the children's behaviour have not provided useful information. Often the distinctions between trait anxiety and state anxiety are ignored. The selection of measurement times should be based on predicted relationships between the pre-measure and the expected effect. Instead, there is little consistency as to when different investigators measure anxiety, thus making comparisons across studies very difficult. Treatment packages often combine so many factors, such as support, coping instructions, information about sensations, that it is next to impossible to evaluate their relative contributions.

THEORETICAL IMPLICATIONS

There is an inadequate empirical base upon which to make predictions regarding the optimal time and manner in which a particular child should be exposed; if at all, to preparatory information. In order to answer this question, it is proposed that an understanding of the factors which influence the individual's set to process information must be obtained. After reviewing the psychological theories regarding the importance of preoperative information, it is apparent that the experimental psychologists who have looked at information and arousal as it effects memory have more to offer than those suggesting a moderate level of arousal facilitates postoperative adjustment. Specifically, the physiological theories of Lacey (1967) and Graham and Clifton (1966) provide a way to evaluate whether the individual is paying attention to the materials being presented.

The most popular psychological theory by Janis (1958) postulated a curvilinear relationship between preoperative anxiety levels and postoperative recovery. The theory states that a moderate level of anxiety facilitates thoughts and fantasies about the process and outcome of surgery and enables the patient to learn to differentiate among real and imagined problems and pain. Through this 'work of worrying', the patient makes a better postsurgery adjustment. The theory has generated much research, however, the results are far from conclusive. Some of the difficulties arise from the ambiguity with which such terms as 'anxiety' or 'arousal' have been defined. The broad three systems approach which defines anxiety as a construct measurable by somatic, behavioural, and cognitive correlates of the individual (Lang, 1968) has not guided the research in this area. Instead, various investigators have chosen to emphasize one system over another. For example, Janis (1958) used global ratings and retrospective self-reports, and ignored the physiology. Others (Auerbach, 1973) have used paper and pencil personality correlates such as Spielberger's State-Trait Anxiety Questionnaire or Byrne's Repression–Sensitization scale, ignoring behavioural measures. A second problem with these early studies is that 'optimal' has consisted of a *post hoc* interpretation based on the consequences of the postoperative behaviour.

Very few studies have attempted to apply the theory to children. Johnson *et al.* (1975) found that sensory information provided for children prior to the removal of a cast did reduce their stress as measured by pulse rate and observed signs of distress, as compared with a taped message about general procedures or a control group receiving no instruction. Presumptions were made regarding the mechanism by which the sensation information might help the children form accurate expectations about what would occur. No measure of information was obtained.

In another study which attempted a more direct investigation of the defence mechanisms involved (Burstein and Meichenbaum, 1979), children were compared for relative preference for hospital-relevant or non-relevant toys one week prior to, immediately after, and one week following surgery. The study makes use of correlations between measures of anxiety and ratings of defensiveness. The low level of anxiety found in some of the children before hospitalization was marginally associated with a high level of anxiety following hospitalization. This supports Janis' contention. Children rated high in defensiveness spent much less time with stress-relevant toys in the prehospitalization group. Most of the other relationships were not in the predicted direction. Winnett (1979) also found that highly defensive child patients did have an absence of anxiety prior to surgery. However, although defensiveness predicted the degree of medically-relevant play, there was no relationship to anxiety reduction postoperatively.

Results of a puppet show therapy for children, five to nine years of age about to have surgery, showed that there was an immediate decrease in Palmar Sweat Index following treatment (Johnson and Stockdale, 1975). However, the night prior to surgery, there was a substantial increase. The authors interpret this as caused by the children's greater knowledge, compared to control patients, about the hospital operative procedures they would encounter. The postsurgery measure did support Janis' theory in that those children who had been exposed to puppet therapy, were less anxious than were control subjects the evening after surgery.

All of these studies made inferences about information being avoided or attended to in children of varying defensiveness. There are objective ways in which the experimenter–therapist can better determine whether the information was processed. Lacey (1967) proposed that the patterns of autonomic responding in a given situation are a reflection of the individual's readiness to receive information from the environment. He and his colleagues have data (Libby et al., 1973) that when the primary task of the situation is to attend, that deceleration in heart rate, accompanied by other sympathetic activation such as vasoconstriction or palmar conductance increase are likely to occur. This fractionation of autonomic response patterns occurs because different tasks require different organizations of the physiology to facilitate different transactions between the organism and the environment. Thus, Lacey considers cardiac deceleration to be something like an instrumental act of the organism, leading to increasing ease of 'environment intake', whereas, cardiac deceleration is likened to a form of rejection of the environment. Graham and Clifton (1966) found evidence within the orienting reflex literature to support this notion. In boys between seven and nine years of age, a decelerative heart rate accompanied by increased respiratory activity occurred with improved analytic task performance (Kagan and Rosman, 1964), reflecting effective information processing.

Therefore, in surgery preparation studies, rather than assume that an increase in heart rate signals anxiety, it is better to study the directional changes of heart rate activity in order to understand whether the individual is likely to take in the information in a given situation. The simultaneous reduction of heart rate and increase in skin conductance would signal that the organism is alert and ready to take information in.

There have been attempts to evaluate preparation effectiveness in terms of cognitive style variables in individuals. These investigations have focused on such classifications as 'avoiders' versus 'copers', 'repressors' versus 'sensitizers', and 'internals' versus 'externals'. The influence of these correlates on ability to utilize preoperative information is not always clear. Andrew (1970) and DeLong (1971) found that 'deniers' showed the poorest recovery from surgery, particularly if they received specific information about the risks of surgery prior to their operations. The locus of control orientation has accounted for individual adjustment with internal-oriented individuals recovering much better from oral surgery (Auerbach *et al.*, 1976). In a different study (Seeman and Evans, 1962) it was found that hospitalized tuberculosis patients classified as internals knew more about their illness and pursued information relevant to it than did those patients classified as externals. Shipley and his colleagues (1978; 1979) were able to explain their data on modelling preparation by analysing the personality correlate of repression–sensitization. Repressors were more anxious with one exposure to preparatory videotape, whereas sensitizers benefited from multiple presentations. Another way to view the individual differences in response style is to study the differences in the autonomic patterns of these learned response styles. It is possible that the relationship between taking in information and rejecting it, is based on the physiological response patterns that underlie these cognitive coping styles. In any event, the personality variables rarely account for much of the variance and it is more useful at this point to examine the general physiological response patterns which facilitate the taking in of information.

FILM MODELLING STUDIES

Our research focus has been on predicting the optimal time and format of presentation of preparatory material to help children adjust to surgery or dental treatment. The contribution of a videotape used for medical preparation was evaluated in terms of whether the children take in the information presented. The practical question of what type of information to present at what time, needs to be restated in terms of the patients' autonomic arousal patterns, age, and previous experience in the feared situation.

In our studies, children were shown preparatory messages preceding their experience with the stressful event (hospitalization or dental treatment). Anticipatory anxiety, reaction to the preparatory message, reaction to the actual stressors, and recovery were measured. The assessment included autonomic activity, self-report, and behaviour. The specific experimental questions were:

1. Does information about impending treatment reduce anxiety, as broadly assessed by co-operative behaviour, sympathetic activation, and self-report of distress?

2. Does information provided through a peer model reduce anxiety more than just giving the information in a demonstration, without a model?
3. Does previous experience attenuate the effectiveness of film modelling?
4. Does the amount of information processed depend upon the age of the child and the pattern of autonomic arousal at the time it is presented?

First we demonstrated that film modelling reduced anxiety in children with no previous hospital experience. Patients were four to twelve years of age, hospitalized for elective surgery. One group saw hospital relevant information depicted through the eyes of a seven-year-old white boy. A group, matched in age, sex, and type of surgery, saw a hospital irrelevant film of a boy going on a fishing trip. The results of this manipulation reflected by the Palmar Sweat Index are illustrated in Figure 1. This measure allows enumeration of the number of active sweat glands, and is a clear index of activity in the sympathetic nervous system. Two findings are of particular interest. First, the immediate effect of viewing the hospital relevant film

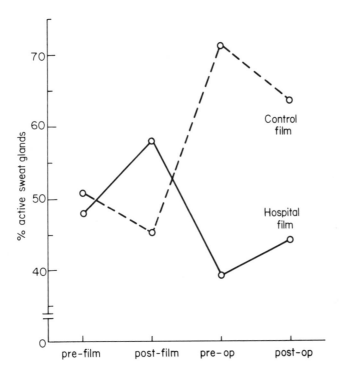

Figure 1. Percentage of active sweat glands for the experimental and control groups across the four measurement periods. Reproduced with permission from Melamed and Siegel, *Journal of Consulting and Clinical Psychology*, **43**, 511–521, 1975

was to significantly raise the level of activation. Secondly, these children showed less sympathetic arousal at the preoperative and postoperative assessments than the control children even though both groups received in-hospital preparation by the staff. Finally, a similar significant finding occurred for self-reported anxiety and observed anxiety-related behaviour. The children who saw the peer modelling film received less pain medication, ate solids more quickly, and reported fewer post-surgery problems (Melamed and Siegel, 1975).

The study of children in the hospital is complicated by multiple contacts with health professionals, different physician preferences regarding pre-medication, and specific differences in medical procedures undertaken. Thus, these same questions were studied in a naturally-controlled laboratory, 'the dental operatory', in which there is sanction for noxious events, a predictable sequence of events (novocaine, cavity preparation, drilling, amalgam placement) and a limited number of professionals involved. Also, since the patient is fairly immobile, concurrent physiological measures can be obtained. In addition, patients return for subsequent treatment; thus, providing a setting in which the learning effects of experience can be evaluated.

First, the previous finding for the effectiveness of a film model on four to eleven

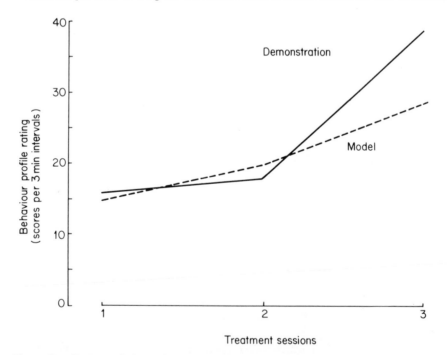

Figure 2.   Degree of disruptiveness during dental treatment and type of videotape preparation. Reproduced with permission from Melamed *et al.*, *Journal of Consulting and Clinical Psychology*, **46**, 1357–1367, 1978

year old children, with no prior experience in the stress situation, was replicated. Again, children showed a significant increase in palmar sweat activity immediately after exposure to the film. Post-treatment reduction of sweating was concordant with ratings of co-operation and reduced disruptiveness obtained by the dentist and an independent observer in children who viewed modelling film as compared to those seeing a control film (Melamed *et al.*, 1975).

Next, the issue of whether peer modelling would be better than presenting the information via a demonstration was studied. A demonstration videotape with the dentist explaining the procedure without a child in the dental chair was devised. There were 80 children, aged four to eleven years, with and without prior dental experience, who viewed either the peer model or demonstration videotape prior to restorative treatment. Peer modelling was more effective in reducing anxiety than the dentist merely providing information about what would occur. Figure 2 illustrates that viewing another child, resulted in fewer disruptive responses than merely observing the demonstration. Self-reports of fear were also lower after observing a peer model, than after a demonstration (Melamed *et al.*, 1978).

The examination of autonomic response patterns in these groups, sheds light on the possible mechanism responsible for the advantage of peer modelling. The Palmar Sweat Index showed a pre-postfilm increase, regardless of which videotape was viewed. This activation is expected under conditions in which relevant information is presented about an anticipated unpleasant event. However, significant differences occurred between heart rate changes in response to the two types of presentations (demonstration versus peer modelling). Figure 3 shows that there was greater deceleration in children watching the injection segment via the peer model, as compared to children viewing a demonstration tape. This finding is consistent with Lacey's hypothesis that cardiac deceleration reflects taking in of information from the environment.

The increase in sweat gland activity is associated only with sympathetic activation, and would be found in any situation (intake or rejection) that prompted individuals to be alert or aroused. Thus, it is only by examining the fractionation of arousal (cardiac deceleration, accompanied by sweat gland activity) that we find both an alert subject, and one capable of taking in information from the environment. It seems plausible then, that subjects watching the demonstration were sympathetically aroused, but not functionally attentive and thus, did not learn what they needed to know to cope with the medical environment; whereas, the subjects who watched the peer model were functionally aroused, and able to process the information necessary in learning what to expect and how to behave. In support of this, it was found that those children viewing peer models recalled more of the information that had been presented than those seeing the demonstration.

Regarding the question of the attenuation of modelling effects in children with previous experience, it makes sense to assume that children with previous experience in a stressful situation already have information about what to expect. This may predispose them to be more or less anxious, depending upon the nature of that

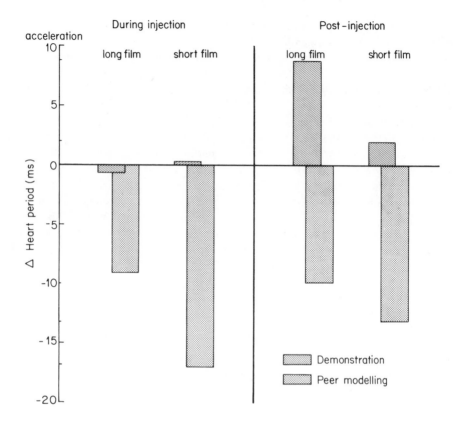

Figure 3.   Change in heart period during the viewing of injection and post-injection
segments of peer modelling or demonstration videotape

previous experience. Peer modelling could provide them with more adaptive coping
techniques, but only if the individual pays attention to the videotape. Our study and
that of Klorman *et al.* (1980) found a failure of modelling, whether it be mastery or
coping, to improve the co-operative behaviour of children who had already had
previous dental treatment, as compared to those previously experienced who
observed a control film treatment. It is imperative also to understand what
differences in autonomic patterning may exist in the child with previous experience
which may enhance or interfere with the acquisition of new information about how
to cope.

To illustrate this point, we examined the surgery preparation of children who
received peer modelling exposure prior to their second operation (Melamed and
Siegel, 1980). These 'experienced' children were at a higher level of sympathetic
arousal and reported a greater number of medical concerns than children viewing
the film prior to their first hospital experience. The peer modelling film was no more

effective than an unrelated film in reducing anxiety in arousal, self-report, or anxiety-related behaviour. Figure 4 compares the second timers with naïve patients on the Palmar Sweat Index at critical points during the hospital experience. It may be seen (lower half of figure) that with inexperienced children, the observation of a peer modelling film reduced arousal as compared with those viewing an unrelated film. However, no such effect occurred when a group of children coming to the hospital for the second operation were compared following either the peer modelling film or an unrelated control film (upper half of figure). To account for the difference, it should be noted that their prefilm levels of sweat gland activity were higher than those of inexperienced children. There were no significant reductions at preoperative or postoperative assessments. These youngsters may have been too aroused sympathetically to take in the information presented. Their previous hospitalization could have led to a sensitization when they were again exposed to the relevant stimuli through the film. Such conditioned emotional arousal should prompt Lacey's 'set of environmental rejection'. It may then be hypothesized that poorer coping in the hospital is attributable to the patient's having obtained less relevant information from the videotape. This hypothesis could be tested if data were available regarding heart rate during the film and an accurate assessment was made of what information the patients had actually acquired.

In a current study at the University of Florida, this question is being examined in detail. Specific hospital relevant material is presented to children while prefilm heart

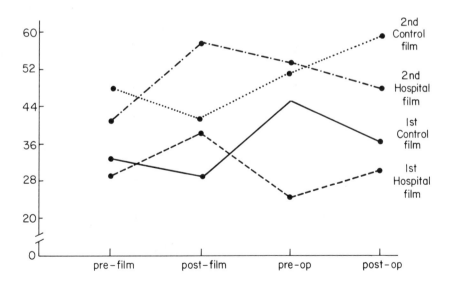

Figure 4. Percentage of active sweat glands for the experimental and control groups across the four measurement periods in children having their first or second operations

rate and sweat activity are recorded. Preliminary findings based on the first fifteen patients support Lacey's hypothesis.

Table 1 summarizes the major population characteristics of these children, who were hospitalized at Shands Teaching Hospital of the University of Florida, Gainesville. Although the range of surgeries is very wide, each child required inpatient hospitalization and general anaesthesia. Effects of previous experience can not yet be evaluated due to the small sample.

Table 1.   Major population characteristics

Age	Previous experience	Type of surgery	Sex	Race
6	No	Hydroureter	M	W
7	No	Cabitus varus of left elbow	M	W
7	No	Aortic stenosis	F	NW
7	Yes	Umbilical hernia	F	NW
7	Yes	Hernia	M	NW
9	No	Femeral anteversion	F	W
10	Yes	Tonsillectomy	M	W
10	Yes	Catheterization of aorta	M	W
10	No	Rectal mass	M	NW
10	No	Urinary tract	M	W
10	Yes	Hernia	M	W
10	Yes	Heart valve closure	M	NW
11	Yes	Renal staghorn calculous	M	W
15	Yes	Congenital scoliosis	F	W
15	Yes	Urinary retention	M	W

Each child was seen individually the night before their scheduled surgery. At this time, many of the preoperative procedures, including blood tests and X-rays had been completed. The patient education specialist informed the child that he/she would have an opportunity to view a slide-audiotape presentation showing what occurs before and after their operation.

'You're going to have an operation' depicts several children of different races, sexes, and ages, describing the procedures and equipment they were exposed to. It has a reassuring theme.*

Several measures were developed to assess the child's perceptions about the operation and a multiple choice test was devised to quantify the amount of information retained after viewing the slide-audiotape material. Such questions include:

1. The shot you get before your operation:
   (a) will sting
   (b) will keep you awake.

* This material was developed by Natalie Small, Ed.D., and is available from the Learning Resources Center, University of Florida, Gainesville, Florida, 32610.

2. NPO means:
   (a) you can't have anything to eat or drink,
   (b) no parents allowed.

Prior to the presentation of the slide tape show, the child's pulse rate was recorded and a plastic impression of sweat gland activity (Johnson and Dabbs, 1967) was obtained. The Hospital Fears Rating Scale was read aloud to the children in order to obtain a self-report of their medical concerns. An independent observer rated the frequency of verbal and non-verbal anxiety behaviours on the Observer Rating Scale of Anxiety. The same measures were re-assessed immediately following the film viewing. Although the parents were given the opportunity to view the slide-tape at another time, they were not present at the time of the children's exposure to the film.

The preliminary results for the small sample size are encouraging as they support the main hypothesis regarding the relationship between individual's autonomic patterning of responses and amount of information acquired through the preparation. The correlation matrix presented in Table 2 shows those relationships relevant to the hypothesis.

Table 2.   Intercorrelations between measures of autonomic arousal, self-report of hospital fears, age, and percentage of information

	Percentage information	Hospital fears
Prefilm heart rate	−0.23	0.002
Postfilm heart rate	−0.31	0.09
Prefilm Palmar Sweat Index	0.52*	−0.52*
Postfilm Palmar Sweat Index	0.10	−0.26
Age	0.758†	−0.32
Hospital Fears Rating Scale	−0.51*	

* $p < 0.07$
† $p < 0.001$

The finding that the higher the prefilm level of sweat gland activity, the greater the per cent of information retained, supported the hypothesis that in order to process information, the patient's nervous system has to be sufficiently sympathetically activated. The direction of the heart rate is also consistent with the prediction that cardiac deceleration facilitates the taking in of information. In both the prefilm and postfilm assessment, lower heart rate levels were associated with greater acquisition of information. It is interesting to note that individuals with high self-reports of anxiety retained less information. These individuals with higher medical concerns also tended to have lower levels of sweat gland activity. Perhaps this apparent discordance between the physiology and the subjective report underlies the mechanism which interferes with the patient's acquisition of relevant information. The individual is not set to attend to the information being provided. There is insufficient activation to promote orienting to the film.

Age also affects a child's readiness to process information. It has been found in previous research in our laboratory (Melamed *et al.*, 1976) that children under the age of seven reported higher medical concerns and showed much greater levels of sweat gland activity if they were shown the preparatory film five to nine days in advance of hospital admission. In the dental study (Melamed *et al.*, 1978) children between the ages of six and eight years, benefited most from modelling presentation. Ferguson (1980) reported that children six to seven years of age benefited from advanced preparation. In the current research, the age of the child correlated most highly with the amount of information retained from the slide tape preparation. There were, however, more children with previous experience in the older age group. The information test may be biased by developmental age considerations.

It would be premature to draw too many conclusions based on the data presented thus far. It is clear, however, that we need to consider not only the type of preparatory materials, but also whether the observer is properly attuned to receive this information. The results do suggest that the autonomic patterns of response are associated with the amount of information retained by children exposed to advanced preparations. Our research suggested that if the patients showed cardiac deceleration in response to the presentation of material, it was more likely that the desired behavioural response was facilitated. This does appear to be mediated by more of the information actually being processed. The initial level of sympathetic arousal, as reflected by Palmar Sweat Index, does seem to have a modulating role in that patients with a higher level of sympathetic activation at the time of film viewing and immediately after, appear to be more alert and retain more information.

The presence of the symbolic peer may have enhanced the child's attention to the relevant information. This received support when viewed within Lacey's theory in that children showed greater heart rate deceleration to a peer model than to a demonstration videotape.

It seems clear that one should not focus solely on what to include in treatment packages, but one must also view preparation as a transaction between an individual and his/her environmental context. Further parametric investigations are needed to define the relationships between individual's patterns of autonomic responsivity and the processing of information relevant to coping with stress.

ACKNOWLEDGEMENTS

I wish to acknowledge the support of the National Institute of Dental Research through grant DE-05305 awarded to the first author. The combined research efforts of Rochelle Robbins, Jesus Fernandez, and Stephanie Smith are reflected in these investigations. The contributions of Drs James Talbert, Bradely Rogers, Farhot Moazam, Dixon Walker, who participated as surgeons; Dr Shirley Graves served as director of pediatric anaesthesiology; Natalie Small, and Patricia Cluff, pediatric patient educators, are gratefully acknowledged. Hospital and nursing staff of pediatric surgery units at Shands Teaching Hospital supported the research effort.

REFERENCES

Andrew, J. (1970) Recovery from surgery, with and without preparatory instruction for three coping styles. *Journal of Personality and Social Psychology*, **15**, 223–226.

Auerbach, S. M. (1973) Trait-state anxiety and adjustment to surgery. *Journal of Consulting and Clinical Psychology*, **40**, 264–271.

Auerbach, S. M., Kendall, P. C., Cuttler, H. F., and Levitt, N. R. (1976) Anxiety, locus of control, type of preparatory information, and adjustment to dental surgery. *Journal of Consulting and Clinical Psychology*, **44**, 809–818.

Burstein, S., and Meichenbaum, D. (1979) The work of worrying in children undergoing surgery. *Journal of Abnormal Child Psychology*, **7**, 121–132.

DeLong, R. (1971) Individual differences in patterns of anxiety arousal, stress relevant information and recovery from surgery. Unpublished doctoral dissertation, University of California, Los Angeles, 1970. *Dissertation Abstracts International*, **32**, 554B.

Ferguson, B. F. (1979) Preparing young children for hospitalization: A comparison of two methods. *Pediatrics*, **64**, 656–663.

Graham, F. K., and Clifton, R. K. (1966) Heart rate change as a component of the orienting response. *Psychological Bulletin*, **65**, 305–320.

Janis, I. L. (1958) *Psychological Stress*, Wiley, New York.

Johnson, J., and Dabbs, J. (1967) Enumeration of active sweat glands. *Nursing Research*, **16**, 273–276.

Johnson, J. E., Kirchhoff, K., and Endress, M. P. (1975) Altering children's distress behavior during orthopedic cast removal. *Nursing Research*, **24**, 404–410.

Johnson, J. E., and Stockdale, D. (1975) Effects of puppet therapy on Palmar sweating of hospitalized children. *John Hopkins Medical Journal*, **137**, 1–5.

Kagan, J., and Rosman, B. L. (1964) Cardiac and respiratory correlates of attention and an analytic attitude. *Journal of Experimental Child Psychology*, **1**, 50–63.

Klorman, R., Hilpert, P., Michael, R., LaGana, C., and Sveen, O. (1980) Effects of coping and mastery modeling. *Behavior Therapy*, **11**, 156–169.

Lacey, J. (1967) Somatic response patterning and stress, in Appley, M., and Trumbull, R. (eds.) *Psychological stress: Issues in Research*. Appleton-Century-Crofts, New York, 14–42.

Lang, P. J. (1968) Fear reduction and fear behavior: Problems in treating a construct, in Shlien, J. (ed.) *Research in Psychotherapy*, American Psychological Association, Washington, D.C. Vol. 3, 90–103.

Libby, W., Jr., Lacey, B. C., and Lacey, J. (1973) Pupillary and Cardiac activity during visual attention. *Psychophysiology*, **10**, 270–294.

Melamed, B. G. (1977) Psychological Preparation for hospitalization, in Rachman, S. J. (ed.), *Contributions in Medical Psychology*, Pergamon Press, Oxford. Vol. 1, 43–74.

Melamed, B. G., and Siegel, L. J. (1975) Reduction of anxiety in children facing hospitalization and surgery by use of film modelling. *Journal of Consulting and Clinical Psychology*, **43**, 511–521.

Melamed, B. G., and Siegel, L. J. (1980) *Behavioral medicine: Practical applications in health care*. Springer Publishing, New York.

Melamed, B. G., Hawes, R., Heiby, E., and Glick, J. (1975) The use of film modeling to reduce uncooperative behavior of children during dental treatment. *Journal of Dental Research*, **54**, 797–801.

Melamed, B. G., Meyer, R., Gee, C., and Soule, L. (1976) The influence of time and type of preparation on children's adjustment to hospitalization. *Journal of Pediatric Psychology*, **1**, 31–37.

Melamed, B. G., Yurcheson, R., Fleece, E., Hutcherson, S., and Hawes, R. (1978) Effects of film modeling on the reduction of anxiety-related behaviors in individuals varying in level of previous experience in the stress situation. *Journal of Consulting and Clinical Psychology*, **46**, 1357–1367.

Peterson, L., and Ridley-Johnson, R. (1980) Pediatric hospital response to surgery on prehospital preparation for children. *Journal of Pediatric Psychology*, **5**, 1–7.

Seeman, M., and Evans, J. W. (1962) Alienation and learning in a hospital setting. *American Sociological Review*, **27**, 772–783.

Shipley, R. H., Butt, J. H., Horwitz, B., and Farbry, J. E. (1978) Preparation for a stressful medical procedure: Effect of amount of stimulus pre-exposure and coping style. *Journal of Consulting and Clinical Psychology*, **46**, 499–507.

Shipley, R. H., Butt, J. H., and Horwitz, B. (1979) Preparation to re-experience a stressful medical examination: Effect of repetitious videotape exposure and copying style. *Journal of Consulting and Clinical Psychology*, **47**, 485–492.

Winnett, R. (1979) *The effect of modeling and play therapy techniques on children's adjustment to brief hospitalization.* Unpublished masters thesis, University of Montana.

20. ASSERTIVENESS TRAINING IN CHILDREN: A COMPARATIVE STUDY OF ROLE PLAY WITH VIDEO-FEEDBACK, ROLE PLAY WITHOUT VIDEO-FEEDBACK, AND DISCUSSION

Gabriele Borrmann, Cornelia Schimikowski, and Irmela Florin

Severe deficiencies of social skills in children may result in excessive dependency, withdrawal, or aggressiveness. Furthermore, juvenile delinquency (Roff *et al.*, 1972), mental health problems (Cowen *et al.*, 1973) and psychosomatic disorders (Mathé and Knapp, 1971) as well as social adjustment problems (Kagan and Moss, 1962) in adulthood have been found to be related to socially maladapted behaviour in childhood. Therefore, it can be assumed that the training of socially competent behaviour in children is of considerable therapeutic and preventive value. Nevertheless, systematic studies comparing the effectiveness of various assertion training procedures in children are scarce (van Hasselt *et al.*, 1979). So far, research has concentrated upon assertiveness training strategies in adolescents and adults. In these studies the relative effectiveness of various over-all training packages as discussion of assertive behavioural alternatives versus rehearsal of assertive behaviour, as well as of training components (instructions, modelling, role-play, video-feedback) has been tested (Eisler *et al.*, 1973; McFall and Twentyman, 1973; Melnick, 1973; Gormally *et al.*, 1975). But it is far from clear to what degree training methods successfully applied with adults are of value in training children. The present comparative group study aimed at helping to close this information gap.

METHOD

Design

The short- and long-term effects of three treatment conditions i.e. role play of assertive behaviour plus video-feedback (Group E_1); role play of assertive behaviour without video-feedback (Group E_2); discussion of assertive behaviour (Group E_3); and one control procedure i.e. placebo role play (Group C), on child behaviour during role play scenes containing *demand behaviour* (target scenes) and others

219

containing *rejection behaviour* (generalization scenes) were tested. After the pre-test the subjects were divided into the four groups which were comparable in pre-test behaviour scores, age, and sex distribution. These groups were then randomly assigned to either one of the three experimental conditions or a control condition. The comparison was made by the use of analysis of variance for repeated measurements on one factor and the application of Newman–Keuls test.

Subjects

Subjects were 44 children (34 boys and ten girls) of nine to 15 years old (mean = 12.5), living in children's homes. They had spent an average of 53 months in such homes, 20 of them had been transferred from one home to another at least once. All but three of them attended special schools for teaching disabled children. All subjects participated voluntarily in the study. They first had been invited to make video recordings of their playmates, be filmed themselves, and to look at the recordings afterwards. This procedure was aimed mainly at their overcoming possible fears of the technical equipment, of being filmed, and of getting video-feedback on their appearances and behaviours. It was also hoped that the children, through their familiarization with equipment and training personnel, would enjoy the participation in the training, and they were only asked to participate when this first step seemed to have been achieved. All but three of the original sample of 47 consented.

Instruments

Role play scenes Role play scenes were designed to contain either demand behaviour or rejection behaviour. In order to get a sample of scenes relevant for home children at the age level of our population, ten children and three educators of a home comparable in structure thought out 38 scenes they found relevant for training; 33 children again from another home, comparable in age and sex distribution, then rated those scenes by means of a four-point scale of the difficulty they may present and inassertiveness they may produce 'in a shy child of their own age'. Each scene was given an inassertiveness score representing the mean rating of the 33 children. Some 24 scenes which were not too similar in content and which did not involve more than two persons were finally selected. Six scenes i.e., three containing demand behaviour and three containing rejection behaviour with comparable inassertiveness scores, were reserved for pre-test, post-test, and follow-up. The others served for training purposes only.

Behavioural ratings
1. Two independent and trained observers rated child behaviour during each test role play situation (at pre-test, post-test, and follow-up) from video-recordings. Every 10 s the video tape was stopped and rating scores were assigned using a

six-point-scale (1 = very inassertive; 6 = very assertive) for each of the following categories: eye contact, other non-verbal behaviour (body posture, facial expression, gestures), loudness of voice, speech fluency, and over-all assertiveness. An assertive behaviour score per child and scene was obtained by calculating the mean rating over intervals and categories as well as over raters. Inter-rater reliability over intervals and categories was 0.92.

2. The four pre- and post-test role play scenes of each child were shown in random order to 21 untrained observers who were first year psychology students and who attributed them to the pre- or post-test condition. As the attributions might have been performed in a stereotypic manner by looking at the content of the scenes only, the raters were misleadingly informed that 50% of those scenes identical in content had been role played at pre-test and the other half at post-test.

Subjective measures

1. The children's anxiety test (KAT). This is a global measure of fears in children containing 19 items and was used in order to reveal possible differential effects of the different training strategies on high versus low anxiety children.

2. The training motivation questionnaire consisted of three questions and was developed and applied in order to obtain feedback on the following items. How content were the children with their role play? How much did they enjoy the sessions? How much did they feel the trainers enjoyed the training? The children rated these questions by means of a four-point rating scale. Besides reflecting the child's motivation to participate in the training, the questionnaire was aimed at reminding the trainers to be enthused in a comparable way throughout all phases of the experiment and in all training conditions.

Procedure

Each child individually participated in a pre-test session lasting for 10 min, two training sessions of 30 min duration each, and a follow-up session of 10 min. Evaluation was conducted at pre-test, post-test, and follow-up. Behaviour ratings was taken from video records for one target and one generalization scene. At the end of each session, the Training Motivation Questionnaire was also completed, while the Children's Anxiety Test (KAT) was given at the first training session.

In each session the child was invited to role play scenes with one of the two trainers serving alternatively as their partners. The content of the scenes to be played was described to the children in a standardized way. That is, the two scenes played in pre-test were described as follows:

Scene 1, demand behaviour: 'You have just bought a ruled writing pad. Leaving the shop you notice that the saleslady has sold you an unruled pad. You walk up to the saleslady and tell her that you want to have the pad exchanged and explain to her why.'

Scene 2, rejection behaviour: 'You have just finished your homework and now want to go cycling. At this moment your friend enters your room and asks, whether he can borrow the bicycle. You tell him, that right now you would like to use it yourself, but that in an hour from now he can borrow it from you.'

For the pre-test, each child was asked to role play, with one of the trainers as a partner, one scene containing *demand behaviour* and a second one containing *rejection behaviour*. Role play was video-recorded and the children were allowed to look at the tape afterwards. At the end of the second training session (post-test) and at follow-up (five weeks later) the children of all groups were asked to role play again two new standardized role play scenes.

Treatment

The treatment of each group was as follow. Group E_1 (Role play plus instructions plus differential reinforcement plus video-feedback): Two scenes requiring demand behaviour were played twice each session. Before role play began the child was told that assertive people differ from shy ones in that they (1) speak up and pronounce clearly, (2) look at the person they are talking to, and (3) stand upright and do not hide their hands behind their backs. At each role play the child himself chose on which aspect of assertive behaviour he wanted to concentrate in his performance. The two trainers alternated randomly as the child's role play partners. After each performance the child was given differential positive feedback for assertive behaviours and in addition was shown the video recordings.

Group E_2 (role play plus instructions plus differential reinforcement. Training in this group differed from training in group E_1 in that the children received no video-feedback.

Group E_3 (discussion plus differential reinforcement). In each of the two training sessions one trainer discussed with the child, for about 7–8 min, possible characteristics of assertive behaviour in scenes requiring demand behaviour. This discussion was led according to a semistructured discussion guide and was aimed at letting the child himself find those aspects of assertive behaviour that were defined and systematically trained in the two other experimental groups. Pointing out relevant aspects of assertive behaviour was differentially reinforced by the trainer. After the discussion the scene was role played and recorded. After role play the child was given a global positive commentary; no video-feedback was given. This procedure was repeated with the second scene.

Group C (placebo role play). In this control condition the children were invited to role play shopping scenes with the trainers alternating randomly as role play partners. The trainers gave no behaviour-directed instructions and no differential feedback, and they were cautious to show neither demand nor rejection behaviour. Two different shopping scenes were role played twice each in a slightly modified form (e.g. buying wallpaper for the kitchen; buying wallpaper for the children's room) during each session. The trainers pretended to video-tape role plays as the children in this control condition were to get used to being filmed to the same degree as the children in the video-feedback condition. However, no video-feedback was given to them.

RESULTS

Assertive behaviour scores in demand (target) and rejection (generalization) scenes

Two-factor (treatments x testing trials) analysis of variance for repeated measurements (pre- and post-test) on one factor were carried out. The analysis revealed significant interactions between testing trials and treatments (for demand scenes: $F = 5.58$, df 3/40, $p < 0.01$; for rejection scenes: $F = 17.25$, df 3/40, $p < 0.01$). The differences shown confirm our expectations in that assertive behaviour scores increase over periods in the experimental groups but they do not in the control group. While assertive behaviour scores did not differ between groups at pre-test (neither in demand nor in rejection scenes), they did differ at the 1 % level of statistical significance (Newman–Keuls test) between each experimental group and

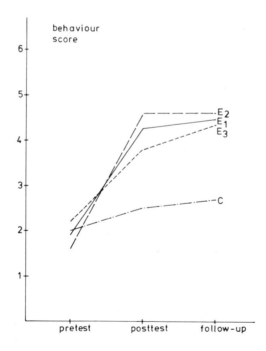

Figure 1.   Mean assertive behaviour scores (demand behaviour) for the four groups at pre-test, post-test, and follow-up condition

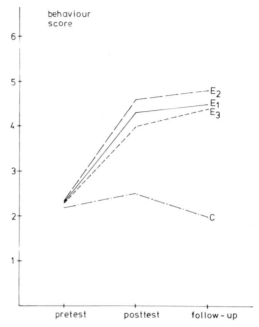

Figure 2.   Mean assertive behaviour scores (rejection behaviour) for the four groups
at pre-test, post-test, and follow-up condition

the control group at post-test. Between the three experimental groups no significant difference existed.

In addition, Newman–Keuls tests over testing trials revealed differences between pre-test and post-test, as well as between pre-test and follow-up to be statistically significant at the 1% level for each of the experimental groups and for demand as well as for rejection scenes (see Figures 1 and 2).

Attribution of role-play scenes (demand and rejection scenes combined) to pre- and post-condition

The synopsis of results of a one-way analysis of variance ($F = 4.6$, df $3/40$, $p < 0.01$) and the Newman–Keuls test showed that role play scenes of the experimental groups were more often correctly attributed to pre- and post-test than the scenes role-played by the control group. While there was no difference in number of correct attributions for the experimental groups, the difference between each experimental group and the control group was significant at the 5% level.

Training motivation

A two-factor analysis of variance for designs with repeated measurements on one factor yielded significant differences between groups in level of motivation ($F = 4.59$, df $3/40$, $p < 0.01$). The Newman–Keuls test showed that group E_1 differed from all other groups at the 5% level from the beginning.

Anxiety level and training effects in the experimental groups

Children with high, medium, and low KAT scores did not differ significantly in the training effect in any of the experimental groups. This was shown by a three-factor analysis of for designs with repeated measurements on one factor (testing trials). Factor 'testing trials' was the only one to prove statistically significant ($F = 211.84$, df $1/24$, $p < 0.01$) and there were no significant interactions between factors.

DISCUSSION

Training in all three experimental conditions led to a significant improvement in assertive behaviour in the target as well as in the generalization role play scenes. Moreover, all experimental conditions proved to be superior to the control condition in these respects. These over-all findings—as well as the finding that the training effects in the experimental groups were fully maintained at follow-up after five weeks—are in accordance with our expectations. We had assumed that focusing on specific components of assertive behaviour—be it during active role play of specific social situations or be it just in discussing how to behave assertively in these same situations—would lead to improved assertiveness. However, mere role play of social scenes, without particular emphasis on assertive behaviour categories, was not expected to yield any improvement.

For the two experimental groups with active role play (E_1, E_2) the results of our study are in line with the findings of some recently conducted single case studies (Beck, et al., 1978; Bornstein et al., 1981). In these, too, it was demonstrated that the active training of assertive behaviour, including behaviour-directed instructions and differential reinforcement of target behaviour, was successful in building up assertive responses.

Discussion strategies, on the other hand, have not been used with children so far. However, Sarason and Ganzer (1973) showed that discussion of assertive behaviour was effective in building up adequate social reactions in juvenile delinquents. As almost all the children of our sample were learning disabled we had assumed that they might find it more difficutl to verbally describe (and then retain for practice) the assertive behaviour components than to train them actively. Contrary to our expectations, the data suggest that discussion of assertive behaviour components is not less effective—even in learning disabled children—than active role play training.

Interestingly, video-feedback did not yield positive effects in addition to active role play training with differential reinforcement. However, studies with adults (Eisler, et al., 1973; Melnick, 1973; Gormally et al., 1975) have not yielded conclusive results in this respect, either.

The children's training motivation remained constant over all phases of the experiment in all four (experimental and control) conditions. This shows that the superiority of the experimental groups over the control group at post-test and follow-up is not due to differences in motivation. This seems noteworthy, since training motivation has almost never been recorded in comparative studies, although it can be assumed that the expectation of different outcome in the groups may differentially influence trainer's motivation and thereby the subjects' motivation.

The sample of children chosen for this study did not show assertiveness deficits of clinical relevance; so, this was an analogue study and one has to be cautious not to generalize the results to clinical populations. However, the data show that the training effects in the experimental groups did not differ between children with high, medium, or low anxiety. Moreover, there was no significant relationship between the time spent in a home and the training effects in the experimental conditions (product-moment-correlation: $r = 0.004$ NS.). And finally, boys and girls did not differ in their training effects obtained as point-biserial correlation between sex and post-test/pre-test difference scores was insignificant ($r = 0.096$). On KAT scores and assertive behaviour scores at pre-test the correlation was $r = 0.13$ NS and the correlation between length of time spent in a home and pre-test assertive behaviour was also insignificant ($r = 0.18$). There was no difference between boys and girls in the assertive behaviour scores at pre-test and it might be assumed that the experimental strategies used in this study can be effectively applied in boys and girls of higher anxiety levels not living in homes. However, testing the generalization of training effects to real-life situations will be a necessary consecutive study.

REFERENCES

Beck, S., Forehand, R., Wells, K. C., and Quante, A. (1978) *Social skills training with children: An examination of generalization from analogue to natural settings.* Unpublished manuscript, University of Georgia.

Bornstein, M., Bellack, A. S., and Hersen, M. (19) Social skills training for highly aggressive children in an inpatient psychiatric setting. *Behavior Modification* (in press) cited in van Hasselt *et al.* 1979.

Cowen, E. L., Pederson, A., Babigian, H., Izzo, L. D., and Trost, M. A. (1973) Long-term follow-up of early detected vulnerable children. *Journal of Consulting and Clinical Psychology*, **41**, 438–446.

Eisler, R. M., Hersen, M., and Agras, W. S. (1973) Effect of video-tape and instructional feedback on non-verbal marital interaction: An analogue study. *Behavior Therapy*, **4**, 551–558.

Gormally, J., Hill, C. E., Otis, M., and Rainey, L. (1975) A microtraining approach to assertion training. *Journal of Counseling Psychology*, **22**, 299–303.

Kagan, J., and Moss, H. A. (1962) *Birth to maturity: A study in social development.* Wiley, New York.

Mathé, A., and Knapp, P. H. (1971) Emotional and adrenal reactions to stress in bronchial asthma. *Psychosomatic Medicine*, **33**, 323–340.

McFall, R. M., and Twentyman, C. T. (1973) Four experiments on the relative contributions of rehearsal, modeling and coaching to assertion training. *Journal of Abnormal Psychology*, **81**, 199–218.

Melnick, J. (1973) A comparison of replication techniques in the modification of minimal dating behavior. *Journal of Abnormal Psychology*, **81**, 51–59.

Roff, M., Sells, B., and Golden, M. (1972) *Social adjustment and personality development in children*. University of Minnesota Press, Minneapolis.

Sarason, I. G., and Ganzer, V. J. (1973) Modeling and group discussion in the rehabilitation of juvenile delinquents. *Journal of Counseling Psychology*, **20**, 442–449.

Van Hasselt, V. B., Hersen, M., Whitehill, M. B., and Bellack, A. S. (1979) Social skill assessment and training for children: an evaluative review. *Behaviour Research and Therapy*, **17**, 413–437.

VI.   MISCELLANEOUS

Learning Theory Approaches to Psychiatry
Edited by John Boulougouris
© 1982 John Wiley & Sons Ltd

21. STRESS AND STRESS-REDUCING FACTORS IN DEPRESSION: A REINFORCEMENT-ORIENTATED ANALYSIS

Lilian Bloeschl

Today, there is widespread agreement in psychiatry and clinical psychology that, within the complex interplay of biological and psychological factors involved in the development of depressive disorder, the role of stressful life events and life conditions may often be of considerable importance (Goodwin and Bunney, 1973; Akiskal and McKinney, 1975). Among the different kinds of psychosocial stressors associated hypothetically with the origin and the maintaining of depression, losses of social relationships and interactions with the environment are particularly prominent. Data related to such a point of view come from several areas of empirical research. First, studies from life-events research, from research on separation and bereavement in humans, and from experimental research on separation in animals (Parkes, 1972; Paykel, 1973; Harlow and Suomi, 1974) have shown that social losses and exit events precede depressive episodes with remarkably high frequency. Second, research within the framework of social psychiatry and behaviourally-orientated clinical psychology (Weissman and Paykel, 1974; MacPhillamy and Lewinsohn 1974; Bloeschl, 1976) has shown that the environmental interactions of depressed persons are characterized by deficiencies and restrictions on the social and the non-social level. Despite numerous methodological difficulties and many unanswered questions, the results of these studies, taken in their totality, seem to provide support for the assumption that losses and deficits of positive interactions with the environment may play a prominent role in the development of depressive response patterns.

Within the clinical–behavioural approach to depression advanced by Ferster (1973) and Lewinsohn (1974) the data cited above are integrated in the concept of loss and deficit of reinforcement. On the basis of this concept, major losses, and reductions of response-contingent positive reinforcers, e.g. by separation loss of occupation, and other psychosocial changes, are seen as important agents eliciting and maintaining depressive reactions. Accordingly, the environment of the depressive client is assumed to be characterized by substantial deficits of positively reinforcing events, particularly but not exclusively of a social kind. These losses and deficits lead, on the one hand, to immediate negative responses on the emotional and the somatic level (dysphoric mood, sleep and eating disturbances, etc.). On the other hand, they lead, by way of extinction, to the decrement of the behavioural repertoire of the individual which appears as a form of passivity and apathy to be one of the most striking features of depressive disorder.

In addition to these two essential aspects, there is a third one which must not be overlooked. It relates to the potential interfering effects of positive reinforcers, i.e. to their potential stress-reducing and stress-inhibiting function (Bloeschl, 1975, 1978). In the light of this hypothesis, losses and reductions of sources of positive reinforcement are assumed to be not only stressful events in themselves. Simultaneously, such changes often may include the loss and the reduction of protective factors supporting the individual in coping with aversive events and conditions as they exist to a more or less high degree in the life situation of any person. Thereby, the balance between positive and negative components in the life of the individual may be further disturbed. The purpose of this chapter is to contribute a few comments to this problem.

In discussing the stress-reducing function of positively reinforcing events and activities and their potential relevance to the course of depressive disorder, it seems necessary to distinguish between (1) the stress-reducing function of positively reinforcing stimuli with particularly high reinforcer value, and (2) the stress-reducing function of positively reinforcing stimuli related to their attention-eliciting and distracting properties and, by this, to the factor of reinforcer variability.

1. First, a substantial part of the empirical studies investigating the role of separation and bereavement in depression has been concerned with the loss of social relationships characterized by close affectional ties. Considering the learning history of an affectionally close social bond the persons involved in such interactions will usually acquire a high amount of conditioned positive reinforcer value for each other, eventually, as Henderson (1977) has pointed out, on a strong biological-evolutionary base. As findings from experimental work with animals and humans suggest (Bovard, 1959, 1962; Kissel, 1965; Ainsworth and Bell, 1970), the presence of a social stimulus of this kind can, under certain circumstances, act as a powerful inhibitor of stress in aversive situations. Clinically relevant data, supporting the view that the lack of a close attachment may seriously diminish the resistance of the individual to the noxious consequences of aversive life events, are coming from various areas of empirical research. Lowenthal and Haven (1968) have studied the connections between the effects of age-related stress conditions, e.g. loss of role, and the presence of a confidant in elderly persons. They found that the psychosocial stress events investigated led to depressed feelings much more frequently in persons who were lacking such an intimate relationship. In the area of clinical depression, Brown

and Harris (1978) reported data indicating that in women the risk of developing a depressive disorder in the presence of a severe life event or major difficulty was significantly higher if there was no close intimate and confiding relationship available. Finally, the results of studies on bereavement and separation suggest that the development of depressive reactions following a crisis of such kind is connected with the lack of supporting contacts with close relatives (Clayton *et al.*, 1972; Smith, 1975). Of course, the complex question in which way the competing responses called forth by positively reinforcing social bonds are interacting with stress responses to aversive life events is far from being answered. Nevertheless, the discussion of interindividual differences in successfully coping with life stressors obviously should not be restricted to the possibilities of different genetic and psychological predispositions. A careful situational analysis of the amount of support provided by major sources of social reinforcement will often indicate that superficially comparable stress situations actually imply very different conditions for depressed and non-depressed individuals.

2. Although the role of close intimate attachment seems to be a particularly prominent factor in the process of dealing with aversive life events, the influence of positively reinforcing social contacts of a more loose and diffuse kind has not be be underestimated in this context, too. Miller and Ingham (1976) found that not only having a close confidant but also having a number of casual friends and acquaintances appears to afford at least partial protection against depression-related symptoms associated with stressful life conditions. Further results suggesting such inter-relationships come from research with normal probands. Bradburn and Caplovitz (1965) and Bradburn (1969) have shown in their empirical studies that it is possible for a person to be in a state of non-depressed mood and general psychological well-being in a life situation including many negative aspects if there are simultaneously compensatory positive aspects. Frequent positive interactions with the social environment on various levels were found to play a substantial role within these inter-relationships. Probably, the stress-reducing effects of positively reinforcing events have to be seen not only with regard to the stress-reducing properties related to their high emotional value but also with regard to their potential interrupting and distracting functions. This hypothesis is in line with the concepts of 'external inhibition' by Pawlow (1953) and of 'inhibitory conditioning' by Guthrie (1952) as well as with recent development in reinforcement theory emphasizing the relationship between the rewarding and the attention-eliciting function of positive reinforcers (Berlyne, 1969; Fowler, 1971). From such a point of view it seems also possible to take into account the potential stress-reducing effects of non-social reinforcers, e.g. of positively reinforcing activities in the area of work and leisure time. Interestingly, the empirical studies cited earlier include a number of findings indicating that it is not only the frequency and the intensity of positively reinforcing contacts and activities which is reduced in the environmental interactions of depressive patients and emotionally depressed persons but also the variability of these events

(Bradburn, 1969; MacPhillamy and Lewinsohn, 1974; Bloeschl, 1976).

Certainly, this does not imply that the distracting effects of positive reinforcers stemming from loose social interactions and pleasurable activities are expected to be central factors in coping with major life crises. However, in coping with the numerous trivial stressors of everyday life (the 'microstressors' proposed by McLean, 1976), and especially with regard to the repeated symbolic self-representation of aversive stimuli by external or internal verbalization which appears to be an important part of depressive symptomatology (Beck, 1974), an individual lacking sources of interfering stimuli of a positive connotation obviously is in a worse position than an individual with many and multifarious resources of this kind.

According to the current status of research in depression in general, the findings and conclusions outlined above must be seen as tentative. As noted earlier, research in this complex area is loaded with severe methodological difficulties particularly regarding the problem of direction of causality within the interplay of the involved variables. Furthermore, the question of specificity appears to be open at this time. Possibly, the lack of stress-inhibiting social relationships and positive interactions with the environment is of influence not only in depression but in other psychological and physiological disturbances, too. Cassel (1976) has pointed to this possibility with regard to the factor of enhanced susceptibility to a wide variety of somatic disorders. Henderson and his coworkers (Henderson, 1977; Henderson et al., 1978a, b, 1980) have found in their empirical studies that a lack of supporting social bonds, a 'primary group deficiency', is associated with depression as well as with neurotic disturbance in general. It will be the task of future research to carry on with detailed empirical analyses of these important problems.

In any case, there are several conclusions resulting from basic research in this field which should not be neglected in the practical therapeutic work with depressive patients. First, in the behavioural analysis of depression it seems necessary to investigate the presence of aversive components in the life situation of the client simultaneously with the lack of positively reinforcing components in his life situation and to consider their balance carefully. Accordingly, in therapy the combination of interventions aimed at decreasing the aversiveness of stressful events and conditions with interventions aimed at increasing positive social contacts and environmental interactions may often be of considerable importance (Lewinsohn and Amenson, 1978; Bloeschl, 1981). Improving these contacts and interactions by newly arranging partnership and family relations, by training social skills to gain and maintain friendships and acquaintances, and by reinstating positively reinforcing non-social activities of various kind possibly not only removes the heavy burden implied in such deficits in themselves. Additionally, it may help the client to develop more adequate strategies to use and to control sources of support in coping with inevitable life stressors.

To summarize, recent research work suggests that, in the analysis of depression-provoking and depression-maintaining psychosocial conditions, the balance between positive and negative components in the life situation of the client has to be considered in a very specific way. Possibly, certain aversive events represent heavy stressors to certain persons, not because these persons are unable to cope with such events principally but because they are missing substantial sources of support and distraction compared with other individuals. From a therapeutic standpoint, these aspects emphasize further the usefulness of strategies striving to remove deficits of positively reinforcing contacts and activities as they are applied in reinforcement-orientated approaches in behaviour modification of depression.

REFERENCES

Ainsworth, M. D. S., and Bell, S. M. (1970) Attachment, exploration, and separation: Illustrated by the behavior of one-year-olds in a strange situation. *Child Development*, **41**, 49–67.

Akiskal, H. S., and McKinney, W. T., Jr. (1975) Overview of recent research in depression. Integration of ten conceptual models into a comprehensive clinical frame. *Archives of General Psychiatry*, **32**, 285–305.

Beck, A. T. (1974) The development of depression: A cognitive model, in Friedman, R. J., and Katz, M. M. (eds.), *The psychology of depression: Contemporary theory and research*. Wiley, New York, pp. 3–27.

Berlyne, D. E. (1969) The reward-value of indifferent stimulation, in Tapp, J. T. (ed.), *Reinforcement and behavior*. Academic Press, New York, pp. 179–214.

Bloeschl, L. (1975) Verstärkerverlust und depressive Reaktion. *Archiv für Psychologie*, **127**, 51–69.

Bloeschl, L. (1976) Zur intra- und extrafamiliären Kontaktstruktur depressiver Patientinnen. *Psychologische Beiträge*, **18**, 465–480.

Bloeschl, L. (1978) *Psychosoziale Aspekte der Depression. Ein lernpsychologisch-verhaltenstherapeutischer Ansatz*. Huber, Bern.

Bloeschl, L. (ed.) (1981) *Verhaltenstherapie depressiver Reaktionen*. Huber, Bern.

Bovard, E. W. (1959) The effect of social stimuli on the response to stress. *Psychological Review*, **66**, 267–277.

Bovard, E. W. (1962) The balance between negative and positive brain system activity. *Perspectives in Biology and Medicine*, **6**, 116–127.

Bradburn, N. M. (1969) *The structure of psychological well-being*, Aldine, Chicago.

Bradburn, N. M., and Caplovitz, D. (1965) *Reports on happiness*, Aldine, Chicago.

Brown, G. W., and Harris, T. (1978) *Social origins of depression*, Tavistock, London.

Cassel, J. (1976) The contribution of the social environment to host resistance. *American Journal of Epidemiology*, **104**, 107–123.

Clayton, P. J., Halikas, J. A., and Maurice, W. L. (1972) The depression of widowhood. *British Journal of Psychiatry*, **120**, 71–78.

Ferster, C. B. (1973) A functional analysis of depression. *American Psychologist*, **28**, 857–870.

Fowler, H. (1971) Implications of sensory reinforcement, in Glaser, R. (ed.), *The nature of reinforcement*. Academic Press, New York, pp. 151–195.

Goodwin, F. K., and Bunney, W. E., Jr. (1973) A psychobiological approach to affective illness. *Psychiatric Annals*, **3**, 19–53.

Guthrie, E. R. (1952) *The psychology of learning*. (2nd edn.) Harper and Brothers, New York.

Harlow, H. F., and Suomi, S. J. (1974) Induced depression in monkeys. *Behavioral Biology*, **12**, 273–296.

Henderson, S. (1977) The social network, support and neurosis. The function of attachment in adult life. *British Journal of Psychiatry*, **131**, 185–191.

Henderson, S., Byrne, D. G., Duncan-Jones, P., Adcock, S., Scott, R., and Steele, G. P. (1978a) Social bonds in the epidemiology of neurosis: A preliminary communication. *British Journal of Psychiatry*, **132**, 463–466.

Henderson, S., Duncan-Jones, P., McAuley, H., and Ritchie, K. (1978b) The patient's primary group. *British Journal of Psychiatry*, **132**, 74–86.

Henderson, S., Byrne, D. G., Duncan-Jones, P., Scott, R., and Adcock, S. (1980) Social relationships, adversity and neurosis. A study of associations in a general population sample. *British Journal of Psychiatry*, (in press).

Kissel, S. (1965) Stress-reducing properties of social stimuli. *Journal of Personality and Social Psychology*, **2**, 378–384.

Lewinsohn, P. M. (1974) Clinical and theoretical aspects of depression, in Calhoun, K. S., Adams, H. E. and Mitchell, K. M. (eds.), *Innovative methods in psychopathology*. Wiley, New York, pp. 63–120.

Lewinsohn, P. M., and Amenson, C. S. (1978) Some relations between pleasant and unpleasant mood-related events and depression. *Journal of Abnormal Psychology*, **87**, 644–654.

Lowenthal, M., and Haven, C. (1968) Interaction and adaptation: Intimacy as a critical variable. *American Sociological Review*, **33**, 20–30.

MacPhillamy, D. J., and Lewinsohn, P. M. (1974) Depression as a function of levels of desired and obtained pleasure. *Journal of Abnormal Psychology*, **83**, 651–657.

McLean, P. D. (1976) Depression as a specific response to stress, in Sarason, I. G., and Spielberger, Ch. D. (eds.), *Stress and anxiety*. Wiley, New York, pp. 297–323.

Miller, P. McC., and Ingham, J. G. (1976) Friends, confidants and symptoms. *Social Psychiatry*, **11**, 51–58.

Parkes, C. M. (1972) *Bereavement. Studies of grief in adult life*. Tavistock, London.

Pawlow, I. P. (1953) *Ausgewählte Werke*. Akademie-Verlag, Berlin.

Paykel, E. S. (1973) Life events and acute depression, in Soctt, J. P., and Senay, E. C. (eds.), *Separation and depression. Clinical and research aspects*. American Association for the Advancement of Science, Washington, D.C., pp. 215–236.

Smith, W. J. (1975) *The desolation of Dido: Patterns of depression and death anxiety in the adjustment and adaptation behaviors of a sample of variably-aged widows*. Unpublished dissertation Sc. D., Boston University.

Weissman, M. M., and Paykel, E. S. (1974) *The depressed woman: A study of social relationships*. University of Chicago Press, Chicago.

Learning Theory Approaches to Psychiatry
Edited by John Boulougouris
© 1982 John Wiley & Sons Ltd

22. PSYCHOPHARMACOLOGICAL TREATMENT IN OBSESSIVE–COMPULSIVE DISORDERS

Evangelos Garelis

Obsessive–compulsive neurosis (OCN) is believed to be a chronic, incapacitating, treatment-resistant disorder. It is not, therefore, surprising that practically all classes of modern psychotropic agents have at times been tried in its treatment.

In attempting to review studies in this field, clear evaluation criteria have to be established. In a similar discussion, Cobb (1977) sets out the characteristics of the 'perfect' treatment study. They include: diagnostic purity, representative sample of adequate size, careful design, valid, reliable, and appropriate measures, control over non-specific treatment, adequate follow-up, definition of 'outcome'. It is unfortunate that most of the studies on the pharmacotherapy of OCN cannot meet even half of these methodological criteria. This fact should be kept in mind throughout the following overview of the various drug treatments used in obsessive–compulsive disorders.

NEUROLEPTICS

Reports on the use of these drugs in OCN were mainly published in the '50s, before the advent of antidepressants and benzodiazepines (Kalinowsky and Hippius, 1969). Several compounds were tried. Chlorpromazine was found ineffective in reducing obsessive–compulsive symptoms; the only benefit was reduction of tension and anxiety (Trethowan and Scott, 1955). Altschuler (1962), in a placebo-controlled, longitudinal study, claimed good results with massive doses of trifluoperazine in a group of twelve patients. The sample, however, included only three cases of primary OCN, one of which improved significantly. Good results were also reported with haloperidol (O'Regan, 1970) but this finding could not be confirmed (Houssain and Ahad, 1970). Studies with neuroleptics have not been carried out in recent years, but it seems clear that they have no specific effect in OCN. They may be of value when obsessions or compulsions appear as a secondary symptom in schizophrenia.

BENZODIAZEPINES

Probably all patients suffering from OCN have taken a benzodiazepine at some time or other. As each new compound is introduced and tried out in mixed neurotic populations, there are invariably claims of some improvement in obsessive–compulsive symptomatology. This reviewer could not find any convincing evidence supporting such claims and is forced to conclude that benzodiazepines do not influence obsessive–compulsive phenomena *per se*. They can be used for the symptomatic relief of anxiety and insomnia, although some therapists would prefer phenothiazines for this purpose. Recent reviews on benzodiazepines do not include OCN in the indications for these drugs (Committee on the Review of Medicines, 1980).

LITHIUM

The ineffectiveness of lithium salts in OCN is one of the best documented cases in the field, as shown by an evaluation of existing data (Schou, 1979). An interesting observation, even though of a rather different nature, was made in one of the lithium studies. Depressed patients who were lithium responders had high scores on obsessive–compulsive features in MMPI; this may be an important discriminator of antidepressant response to lithium (Donelly *et al.*, 1979).

MAO INHIBITORS

The suggestion that phenelzine improves OCN (Jain *et al.*, 1970) was not followed by any systematic study. Therefore, the effect of MAO inhibitors in OCN remains unknown.

ANTIDEPRESSANTS

Early reports on the effectiveness of antidepressive drugs (Geissmann and Kammerer, 1964; Fernandez and Lopez-Ibor, 1967), induced an impetus of work with these compounds (Table 1). Studies with antidepressants other than

Table 1.   Antidepressive drugs in obsessive–compulsive disorders

Authors	Drugs
Mayer-Gross *et al.*, 1969	Imipramine, amitryptiline, desipramine
Freed *et al.*, 1972	Imipramine, amitryptiline
Ananth *et al.*, 1978	Amitryptiline (versus clomipramine)
Ananth *et al.*, 1975	Doxepin
Väisänen *et al.*, 1977	Mianserin
23 studies (1967–1980)	Clomipramine (CM)

Table 2. Clomipramine in obsessive–compulsive disorders. (Uncontrolled studies)

Study	N	Daily dose (mg)	Duration	Improvement
Studies before 1970 (n = 6, cited by Ananth, 1977)	67	≤400 mg	—	73%
Capstick, 1971, 1975, 1977	33	300 p.o.(+ i.v. in 10)	12 months	70%
Marshall and Micev, 1973, 1975	22	300 i.v./150 p.o.	3–18 months	80%
Collins, 1973 (cited in Beaumont, 1973)	65	250 i.v./450 p.o.	2–6 months	83%
Walter, 1973	10	250 i.v.	3–4 weeks	60–100%
Rack, 1977; Allen and Rack, 1975	28	150 p.o./200 i.v.	3–6 weeks	61%
Waxman, 1975	10	150–225 p.o.	6 weeks	33–47%
Singh et al., 1977	17	175–300 p.o.	4 weeks	60%
Ananth, 1977; Ananth et al., 1979	20	100–300 p.o.	4 weeks	45–95%

clomipramine are generally open trials, without control treatments and were done in small samples with poorly-defined subjects. They generally report significant improvements. In the two controlled studies existing, amitriptiline (Ananth et al., 1978) and nortryptiline (Thorén et al., 1980a) were found inferior to clomipramine.

Clomipramine (CM) has been used very extensively. This is partly due to its availability for intravenous administration, which was thought to be superior to oral treatment. Preliminary reports on this drug were so enthusiastic that some investigators considered CM a specific anti-obsessive agent (Capstick, 1971). The superiority of intravenous over the oral treatment has not been proved (Capstick, 1975). Even though the intravenous method is still practised systematically in some centres (O'Flanagan, 1979), no controlled study has evaluated it, mainly because of ethical reasons. Serious side effects (haemoglobinuria, venous thrombosis, epileptic seizures) have been reported (Rack, 1973; Marshal and Micev, 1973). Most of the uncontrolled studies on CM in the last decade are shown on Table 2. It is difficult to compare these studies, because of great variations in patient selection, measures of outcome, duration of treatment and follow-up. But if the results are evaluated on the dichotomy improved/not improved cases, the over-all estimate is that approximately 70% of about 400 patients benefited from CM treatment.

This percentage would be quite comparable to therapeutic results achieved with behaviour-therapy techniques (Table 1 in Foa and Steketee, 1979). It is obvious, however, that the value of a certain treatment can not be established on open studies alone.

Controlled studies on CM in OCN are quite few (Table 3). Comparison among them also presents many difficulties, because of important methodological differences. Waxman (1977) reported a study on a mixed neurotic population, rated by 19 general practitioners in which 14 patients on CM (150 mg daily) did much better than 19 patients on diazepam after six weeks. But the number of obsessions in the two groups of subjects was very small, thus rendering any statistical evaluation meaningless. Karabanow (1977) studied 20 depressed patients, with obsessive–compulsive and phobic traits, severe enough to require treatment. Following a double blind design, half of the group received CM 100 mg daily and the other half identical placebo for six weeks. Obsessive scores, evaluated on the Beaumont–Seldrup scale diminished gradually from a mean of 44.5 down to 16.1 at

Table 3.　Clomipramine in obsessive–compulsive disorders. (Controlled studies)

Authors	N	Daily dose (mg)	Duration	Control treatment
Waxman, 1977	10	150	6 weeks	Diazepam
Karabanow, 1977	10	100	6 weeks	Placebo
Amin et al., 1977	6	Uncompleted study		Behaviour therapy
Solyom and Sookman, 1977	6	300	6 weeks	Behaviour therapy
Ananth et al., 1978	20	75–300	4 weeks	Amitryptiline
Marks et al., 1980	20	183/145	8 months	Placebo

the end of the treatment. No change was found in the placebo group. The difference was highly significant.

The study by Amin *et al.* (1977) started with the ambitious aim of comparing CM, behaviour therapy, and placebo. But of their twelve patients (six with phobic and six with obsessive–compulsive neurosis), only eight completed the study, thus leaving only one or two cases of OCN in each of the three groups. Therefore, no conclusion can be drawn from this study, although the authors suggest that the combination of CM with behaviour therapy gave the best results. This suggestion is further substantiated by the findings of Solyom and Sookman (1977) in a much better study. Six patients received CM 300 mg daily for six weeks, nine cases were given twice-weekly sessions of flooding for six months, the third group, also of nine patients, was treated for the same period of time by a thought-stopping technique. All subjects in the study were 'pure' obsessive–compulsives. Depressed patients were excluded. Outcome was evaluated by a battery of psychometric tests, including the Leyton Inventory. CM reduced the total obsessive symptomatology by 50%. The drug was as effective as flooding and more effective than thought stopping in reducing ruminative symptoms, but it was considerably less effective than behaviour therapy in reducing compulsions. At one-year follow up, patients who improved on CM showed further improvement on maintenance doses of 75–150 mg daily. There were two full recoveries.

In a four-week double blind study, employing a daily dose of 75–300 mg in 20 patients Ananth *et al.* (1978) found clear superiority of CM over amitryptiline in the treatment of OCN. Complete data of this study have not been published.

In a series of publications (Rachman *et al.*, 1979; Marks *et al.*, 1980; Stern, *et al.*, 1980), the research group at the Institute of Psychiatry in London, reported the results of the most rigorous longitudinal study available. They compared the effect of CM and exposure in a total of 40 patients. The complex design of the study does not allow for firm conclusions on the comparative long-term efficacy of CM treatment versus behaviour therapy. The two treatments seemed to be additive rather than synergistic. CM was significantly better than placebo on nearly all measures of rituals, mood, and social adjustment; the different was maximal after 10–18 weeks.

At one year follow-up, four months after discontinuation of the drugs, CM treated patients were not significantly better than the group who had been given placebo. Improvement on CM was clear only in patients who had high depression scores at the start, suggesting that CM acted more as an antidepressant than as an anti-obsessive agent. This finding agrees with the results of Capstick and Seldrup (1973), and Thorén *et al.* (1980a). Other investigators, however, did find improvement in patients with OCN even in the absence of depression (Solyom and Sookman, 1977).

The London study also provided evidence that a 'therapeutic window' exists in CM treatment of OCN, similar to the one in the treatment of depression. The range of effective plasma levels was 100–250 ng ml^{-1} for clomipramine, and 230–550 ng ml^{-1} for desmethylchlorimipramine, which is thought to be the active metabolite.

OTHER PHARMACOLOGICAL TREATMENTS

In a preliminary study with L-tryptophan in seven patients, considerable improvement was noted after one month of therapy. Doses ranged from 3–9 g daily (Yaryura-Tobias and Bhagavan, 1977).

Rabavilas *et al.* (1979), in the course of a psychophysiological study, found no acute effect of practolol (300 mg daily for three days) in obsessive–compulsive symptomatology in twelve patients.

NEUROCHEMICAL SUBSTRATE

There are several theories on the involvement of biogenic amines in OCN (Ananth, 1976), but very little work has been done in this field. Some evidence in favour of the serotonin hypothesis is given by the finding that the anti-obsessive effect of CM appeared to be correlated with the decrease of 5-HIAA in the cerebrospinal fluid (Thorén *et al.*, 1980b). Also, serotonin was found to be low in the blood of obsessive–compulsives (Neziroglu, 1978).

In conclusion, it can be said that various psychoactive drugs have been used in the treatment of OCN, without proved effectiveness. The antidepressant drug clomipramine has been studied most extensively to date. It is better than placebo and gives satisfactory results particularly in cases where depression is a prominent symptom. High doses for prolonged periods of time are needed to sustain the therapeutic effect. Clomipramine and behaviour therapy have additive and probably complementary effects in depressed obsessive–compulsive patients. A combination of the two treatments is probably indicated in such cases, whereas in 'pure' obsessive–compulsives exposure is the treatment of choice. The comparative effect of other antidepressants and the biochemical substrate in OCN remain unknown at the present time.

REFERENCES

Allen, J. J., and Rach, P. H. (1975) Changes in obsessive/compulsive patients as measured by the Leyton Inventory before and after treatment with clomipramine. *Scottish Medical Journal*, **20, suppl. 1,** 41–44.

Altschuler, M. (1962) Massive doses of trifluoperazine in the treatment of compulsive rituals. *American Journal of Psychiatry*, **119,** 367–368.

Amin, M. M., Ban, T. A., Pecknold, J. C., and Klingner, A. (1977) Clomipramine (Anafranil) and behaviour therapy in obsessive–compulsive and phobic disorders. *Journal of International Medical Research*, **5, suppl. 5,** 33–37.

Ananth, J. (1976) Treatment of obsessive–compulsive neurosis: Pharmacological approach. *Psychosomatics*, **17,** 180–184.

Ananth, J. (1977) Treatment of obsessive–compulsive neurosis with clomipramine (Anafranil). *Journal of International Medical Research*, **5, suppl. 5,** 38–41.

Ananth, J., Pecknold, J. C., Van den Steen, N., and Engelsmann, F. (1978) Chlorimipramine in obsessive–compulsive neurosis: A standard controlled study. *11th CINP Congress*, Vienna (Abstr.).

Ananth, J., Solyom, L., Bryntwick, S., and Krishnappa, U. (1979) Chlorimipramine therapy for obsessive–compulsive neurosis. *American Journal of Psychiatry*, **136**, 700–701.

Ananth, J., Solyom, L., Solyom, C., and Sookman, B. A. (1975) Doxepin in the treatment of obsessive–compulsive neurosis. *Psychosomatics*, **16**, 185–187.

Beaumont, G. (1973) Clomipramine (Anafranil) in the treatment of obsessive–compulsive disorders—A review of the work of Dr G. H. Collins. *Journal of International Medical Research*, **1**, 423–424.

Capstick, N. (1971). Chlorimipramine in obsessional states *Psychosomatics*, **12**, 332–335.

Capstick, N. (1975). Chlomipramine in the treatment of the true obsessional state. *Psychosomatics*, **16**, 21–25.

Capstick, N. (1977) Clinical experience in the treatment of obsessional states. *Journal of International Medical Research*, **5, suppl. 5**, 71–80.

Capstick, N., and Seldrup, J. (1973) Phenomenological aspects of obsessional patients treated with chlomipramine. *British Journal of Psychiatry*, **122**, 719–720.

Cobb, J. (1977) Drugs in treatment of obsessional and phobic disorders with behavioral therapy-possible synergism, in Boulougouris, J. C., and Rabavilas, A. D. (eds.), *The treatment of phobic and obsessive–compulsive disorders*, Pergamon, New York, pp. 127–138.

Committee on the Review of Medicines (1980) Systematic review of the benzodiazepines. *British Medical Journal*, **i**, 910–912.

Donelly, E. F., Murphy, D. L., and Waldman, I. V. (1979) Obsessionalism and response to lithium. *British Medical Journal*, **i**, 1627–1629.

Fernandez, J. and Lopez-Ibor, J. J. (1967) Monochlorimipramine in the treatment of psychiatric patients resistant to other therapies. *Actas Luso-Espaniolas de Neurologia y Psiquiatria*, **26**, 119–147.

Foa, E. B., and Steketee, G. S. (1979) Obsessive–compulsives: Conceptual issues and treatment intervention. *Progress in Behavior modification*, **8**, 1–53.

Freed, A., Kerr, T. A., and Roth, M. (1972) The treatment of obsessional neurosis. *British Journal of Psychiatry*, **120**, 590–591.

Geissmann, P., and Kammerer, T. (1964) L'imipramine dans la névrose obsessionelle. Etude de 30 cas. *Encephale*, **53**, 369–382.

Hussain, M. Z., and Ahad, A. (1970) Treatment of obsessive–compulsive neurosis. *Canadian Medical Association Journal*, **103**, 648–650.

Jain, V. K., Swinson, R. P., and Thomas, J. C. (1970) Phenelzine in obsessional neurosis. *British Journal of Psychiatry*, **117**, 237–238.

Kalinowsky, L. B. and Hippius, H. (1969). *Pharmacological convulsive and other somatic treatments in psychiatry*. Grune and Stratton, New York.

Karabanow, O. (1977) Double-blind controlled study in phobias and obsessions. *Journal of International Medical Research*, **5, suppl. 5**, 42–48.

Marks, I. M., Stern, R. S., Mawson, D., Cobb, J., and McDonald, R. (1980) Clomipramine and exposure for obsessive–compulsive rituals: I. *British Journal of Psychiatry*, **136**, 1–25.

Marshall, W. K., and Micev, V. (1973) Clomipramine (Anafranil) in the treatment of obsessional illness and phobic anxiety states. *Journal of International Medical Research*, **1**, 403–412.

Marshall, W. K., and Micev, V. (1975) The role of intravenous clomipramine in the treatment of obsessional and phobic disorders. *Scottish Medical Journal*, **20**, 49–53.

Mayer-Gross, W., Slater, E., and Roth, M. (1969). *Clinical Psychiatry*, 3rd edn. Baillière, Tindall and Cassell, London.

Neziroglu, F. (1978) A combined behavioral-pharmacotherapy approach to obsessive–compulsive disorders. II. *World Congress of Biological Psychiatry, Barcelona*, Abst.

O'Flanagan, P. M. (1979) Experience with clomipramine (Anafranil) infusion treatment. *British Journal of Clinical Practice*, **3**, 69–71.

O'Regan, J. B. (1970) Treatment of obsessive–compulsive neurosis with haloperidol. *Canadian Medical Association Journal*, **103**, 167–168.

Rabavilas, A. D., Boulougouris, J. C., Perissaki, C., and Stefanis, C. (1979) The effect of peripheral beta-blockade on psychophysiologic responses in obsessional neurotics. *Comprehensive Psychiatry*, **20**, 378–383.

Rachman, S., Cobb, J., Grey, S., McDonald, B., Mawson, D., Sartory, G., and Stern, R. (1979) The behavioural treatment of obsessional–compulsive disorders, with and without clomipramine. *Behaviour Research and Therapy*, **17**, 467–478.

Rack, P. H. (1977) Clinical experience in the treatment of obsessional states. *Journal of International Medical Research*, **5, suppl. 5**, 81–90.

Schou, M. (1979) Lithium in the treatment of other psychiatric and nonpsychiatric disorders. *Archives of General Psychiatry*, **36**, 856–859.

Singh, A. N., Saxena, B., and Gent, M. (1977) Clomipramine (Anafranil) in depressive patients with obsessive neurosis. *Journal of International Medical Research*, **5, suppl. 5**, 25–32.

Solyom, L., and Sookman, D. (1977) A comparison of clomipramine hydrochloride (Anafranil) and behaviour therapy in the treatment of obsessive neurosis. *Journal of International Medical Research*, **5, suppl. 5**, 49–61.

Stern, R. S., Marks, I. M., Mawson, D., and Luscombe, D. K. (1980) Clomipramine and exposure for compulsive rituals: II. Plasma levels side effects and outcome. *British Journal of Psychiatry*, **136**, 161–166.

Thorén, P., Asberg, M., Conholm, B., Jornestedt, L., and Traskman, L. (1980a) Clomipramine treatment of obsessive–compulsive disorder. I. A controlled clinical trial. *Archives of General Psychiatry*, **37**, 1281–1288.

Thorén, P., Åsberg, M., Bertilsson, L., Mellström, B., Sjöqvist, F., and Träskman, L. (1980b). Clomipramine treatment of obsessive–compulsive disorder. II. Biochemical aspects. *Archives of General Psychiatry*, **37**, 1289–1294.

Trethowan, W. H., and Scott, P. A. L. (1955) Chlorpromazine in obsessive–compulsive and allied disorders. *Lancet*, **i**, 781–785.

Väisänen, E., Ranta, P., Nummikko-Pelkonen, A. and Tienari, P. (1977) Mianserin hydrochloride (ORG GB 94) in the treatment of obsessional states. *Journal of International Medical Research*, **5**, 289–291.

Walter, C. J. S. (1973) Clinical impressions on treatment of obsessional states with intravenous clomipramine (Anafranil). *Journal of International Medical Research*, **1**, 413–416.

Waxman, D. (1975) An investigation into the use of Anafranil in phobic and obsessional disorders. *Scottish Medical Journal*, **20**, 61–66.

Waxman, D. (1977) A clinical trial of clomipramine and diazepam in the treatment of phobic and obsessional illness. *Journal of International Medical Research*, **5**, Suppl. 5, 99–110.

Yaryura-Tobias, J. A., and Bhagavan, H. N. (1977) L-Tryptophan in obsessive–compulsive disorders. *American Journal of Psychiatry*, **134**, 1298–1299.

23. IS EMG FEEDBACK TRAINING EFFECTIVE IN THE TREATMENT OF ANXIETY?

Yves Lamontagne, Lawrence Annable, and Yvon-Jacques Lavallée

Biofeedback techniques permit an individual's physiological signal to be recorded, amplified, and transformed into a visual or auditive stimulus; the subject can thus become conscious of an involuntary physiological function and train himself to modify it (Lamontagne, 1976). EMG feedback is perhaps the most useful of all biofeedback instruments (Fuller, 1977), especially in psychiatry (Nigl and Jackson, 1979), and has been applied with some success as a treatment for insomnia (Stoyva, 1975; Lamontagne, 1978a), tension headaches (Budzynski *et al.*, 1970), obsessions (Delk, 1977), drug addiction (Lamontagne *et al.*, 1975), and anxiety (Raskin *et al.*, 1973).

Our group became interested in EMG feedback training in the treatment of anxiety in 1973. After some exploratory studies (Lavallée and Lamontagne, 1974; Lamontagne *et al.*, 1975) we first evaluated the effects of α-wave and EMG feedback training with anxious students who were also drug users (Lamontagne *et al.*, 1977). Some authors had already suggested that biofeedback could help in the treatment of alcohol and drug abuse by inducing either a relaxation response or a modification of the state of consciousness (Davidson and Krippner, 1972; Steffen, 1975). In this experiment 75 students were randomly assigned to five experimental groups: α-wave feedback, EMG feedback, joked feedback, no feedback, and no treatment. All treated subjects participated in twelve 30-minute training sessions, four in the laboratory and eight at their college, over a period of four weeks. Results showed that EMG biofeedback reduced drug use among medium (6–13 times monthly) and heavy users (14 or more times monthly) and decreased their anxiety ratings. Moreover, these effects were largely maintained during a six-month follow-up period. These results tended to suggest that EMG feedback can serve as a means for the prevention of drug abuse, particularly where anxiety is a predisposing factor. They also suggest that this type of training has more to offer than electroencephalographic feedback for the treatment of pathology related to anxiety. α-Wave activity seemed to be much more difficult to control than EMG levels and only those subjects who manifested high α-wave levels at baseline were able to benefit from this type of training.

For these reasons we stopped working with α-wave feedback and we investigated the effects of EMG feedback, diazepam, and their combination on patients suffering from anxiety neurosis (American Psychiatric Association, 1968). In this study, 40 patients were randomly assigned to one of four groups in a 2×2 factorial design: EMG feedback plus diazepam, EMG feedback plus diazepam placebo, EMG control (no feedback) plus diazepam, and EMG control plus diazepam placebo (Lavallée *et al.*, 1977a). During treatment, the effects of EMG feedback plus diazepam were additive in reducing muscular tension. Although all active treatment groups reduced their anxiety after treatment, diazapam-treated subjects (with or without feedback) did less well than other subjects on anxiety measurements, adjuvant medication usage and home practice. The results indicated that EMG feedback treatment had a more prolonged therapeutic effect for chronically anxious patients when it was given without diazepam medication. Nevertheless, although we thought that biofeedback training was beneficial to certain anxious patients, we felt sure that other factors influenced its effectiveness and we believed that the interaction between biofeedback training, relaxation training and various psychotropic drugs needed to be investigated more thoroughly to determine the positive and negative effects of various combinations of these therapeutic modalities. Recently, Raskin *et al.* (1980) compared muscle feedback, transcendental meditation, and relaxation therapy in the treatment of chronic anxiety. There were no differences between treatments with respect to treatment efficacy, onset of symptom amelioration, or maintenance of therapeutic gains. The authors found no evidence suggesting that the degree of muscle relaxation induced by any of the treatments is related to therapeutic outcome. They conclude that relaxation therapies as a sole treatment appear to have a limited place in the treatment of chronic anxiety. It now seems clear to us that EMG feedback offers a means of creating a state of internal tranquillity (Lamontagne, 1979) by reducing the patient's general level of arousal and that it should only be used as an adjunct to behavioural or insight psychotherapy as part of an over-all treatment plan for anxiety.

At the present time, most of the chronic patients in our out-patient clinic start treatment by receiving two or three sessions of autogenic training exercises before beginning EMG feedback and continue to practise relaxation at home at least 20 min a day during treatment and follow-up. We favour autogenic training exercises (Schultz, 1960; Lamontagne, 1978b), rather then progressive relaxation (Jacobson, 1974) because, being a passive method of relaxation like EMG feedback, the patient is already familiar with this type of relaxation when feedback training starts. Furthermore, we think that this procedure helps the patient to avoid becoming dependent on the instrumentation and may motivate him to continue the practice of relaxation as a self-control procedure after treatment. The use of minor tranquillizers is often helpful at the beginning of treatment but the dose is decreased gradually as the patient becomes more familiar with the technique of relaxation. Finally, when anxiety decreases to a tolerable level, behavioural techniques, or psychotherapy are introduced into the treatment plan. The following case summary is a typical example of our procedure.

A young physician of 27 years of age requested treatment for very severe anxiety that had developed five months earlier at the time when he became a hospital registrar. When we saw him, he was taking diazepam 10 mg three times a day and was virtually panic-stricken. His case history revealed that he had a sexual dysfunction problem and had carried out compulsive checking rituals since the age of 16. At the interview, he reported that he wanted treatment only for his anxiety and that he did not want to discuss any other problem. The patient was kept on his regular medication and received two sessions of autogenic training exercises followed by eight sessions of EMG feedback training. After the third session of feedback, it was possible to reduce the dosage of diazepam to 5 mg three times a day and the drug was completely stopped after the sixth session. At the end of the fourth session of feedback the patient was much less anxious and asked if some form of treatment would be possible for his rituals. A programme of response prevention was elaborated and the patient co-operated well. At the seventh feedback session, the patient reported that he felt much better and that the frequency of his rituals had declined from an average of 24 to three times a day. He also reported that he would now be willing to discuss his occasional sexual impotency. Eight sessions of short-term psychotherapy were offered after the feedback sessions to complete the treatment. During these sessions, it became evident that his sexual impotency occurred when he was angry at his girlfriend. His relationship with his girlfriend was examined and he was taught to express his hostility verbally. At the end of treatment (18 sessions), the patient reported that his sexual problem had disappeared, that he continued to practise one or two short rituals a day and felt only mildly anxious from time to time. Tension in the frontalis muscle which had been at 42 μ V before treatment had decreased to 6 μ V. At a three month follow-up, he was living with his girlfriend, still practising relaxation regularly and satisfied with the results of the treatment combination. As can be seen, relaxation and EMG feedback training were not only useful in decreasing anxiety but helped the patient to establish a positive rapport with the therapist and to become more involved in the psychotherapeutic process.

Although this practical treatment plan has been beneficial for many anxious patients, we were interested to know the characteristics of patients who are able to decrease their anxiety by EMG feedback training alone. In our most recent study (Lavallée et al., 1980) which included 32 patients, we found that subjects who reported great improvement in their anxiety after eight EMG feedback training sessions had a significantly ($p < 0.05$) higher mean score for extraversion on the Eysenck Personality Inventory (Eysenck and Eysenck, 1968) and a lower mean score for depression on the Minnesota Multiphasic Personality Inventory (Hathaway and McKinley, 1967) when they entered the study than those who did not report improvement. The results thus indicate that extraverted patients may respond better to feedback training and that signs of depression may be a contraindication for this form of treatment. Other studies evaluating characteristics of patients who respond well to a particular form of treatment are needed to elucidate the types of relaxation training that may most benefit the individual patient.

In conclusion, the days when biofeedback was claimed to be a panacea for all kinds of disorders are now over and it is clear that EMG feedback training may not be more effective than other relaxation techniques (Lavallée *et al.*, 1977b; Raskin *et al.*, 1980). The clinical approach to anxiety must necessarily include an over-all treatment strategy. The therapist must know what the patient wants and take into account differences in intelligence and motivation for treatment. If the patient wants only to alleviate his anxiety or is preoccupied by his symptoms, a combination of drugs, relaxation exercises and EMG feedback training can sometimes be helpful. If the patient is able to look after himself, performs useful work and is independent, the addition of a variety of psychotherapeutic techniques can bring long-lasting results. The patient must be a responsible, co-operative and active participant in his treatment. Finally, the therapist's view of the patient as an impaired person rather than a sick person (Clancy and Noyes, 1979) and his encouragement and enthusiasm can reinforce the patient's self-esteem, self-reliance, and self-confidence. Anxiety being a multifaceted disorder, comparative studies are needed to determine the optimum combination of therapeutic techniques for treatment of its different clinical manifestations.

REFERENCES

American Psychiatric Association (1968) *Diagnostic and statistical manual of mental disorders* (2nd ed.), American Psychiatric Association, Washington.

Budzynski, T., Stoyva, J., and Adler, A. (1970) Feedback induced muscle relaxation: application to tension headaches. *Journal of Behavior Therapy and Experimental Psychiatry*, **1**, 205–211.

Clancy, J., and Noyes, R. (1979) The medical approach to anxiety neurosis. *Psychosomatics*, **20**, 663–667.

Davidson, R., and Krippner, S. (1972) Biofeedback research: the data and their implications, in *Biofeedback and Self-Control*, Aldine-Atherton, Chicago, pp. 3–34.

Delk, J. L. (1977) Use of EMG biofeedback in behavioural treatment of an obsessive–phobic–depressive syndrome. *Diseases of the Nervous System*, **38**, 938–939.

Eysenck, H. J., and Eysenck. S. B. G. (1968) *Manual for the Eysenck Personality Inventory*. Educational and Industrial Testing Service, San Diego.

Fuller. G. D. (1977) *Biofeedback: Methods and procedures in clinical practice*. Biofeedback Press, San Francisco.

Hathaway, S. R., and McKinley, J. C. (1967) *Minnesota Multiphasic Personality Inventory*. The Psychological Corporation, New York.

Huffer, V. (1978) *Biofeedback: The need for a flexible approach*. Paper presented at the 25th Annual Meeting, Academy of Psychosomatic Medicine, Atlanta, November 1978.

Jacobson, E. (1974) *Progressive relaxation*, University of Chicago Press, Chicago.

Lamontagne, Y., Hand, I., Annable, L., and Gagnon, M. A. (1975) Physiological and psychological effects of alpha and EMG feedback training with college drug users: a pilot study. *Canadian Psychiatric Association Journal*, **20**, 337–349.

Lamontagne, Y. (1976) Biofeedback in psychiatry. *Modern Medicine of Canada*, **31**, 762–764.

Lamontagne, Y., Beauséjour, R., Annable, L., and Tétreault, L. (1977) Alpha and EMG feedback training in the prevention of drug abuse. *Canadian Psychiatric Association Journal*, **22**, 301–310.

Lamontagne, Y. (1978a) Treatment of prurigo nodularis by relaxation and EMG feedback training. *Behaviour Analysis and Modification*, **2**, 246–249.

Lamontagne, Y. (1978b) Les techniques de relaxation. *La Vie Médicale au Canada Français*, **7**, 56–65.

Lamontagne, Y. (1979) Our experience on EMG feedback training. *Archives of Greek Association for Behaviour Modification*, **1**, 19–21.

Lavallée, Y. J., and Lamontagne, Y. (1974) Les applications thérapeutiques de la rétroaction biologique. *Union Médicale du Canada*, **103**, 264–271.

Lavallée, Y. J., Lamontagne Y., Pinard, G., Annable, L., and Tétreault, L. (1977a) Effects of EMG feedback, diazepam and their combination on chronic anxiety. *Journal of Psychosomatic Research*, **21**, 65–71.

Lavallée, Y. J., Beausejour, R., Lamontagne, Y., and Annable, L. (1977b) Effets subjectifs de l'entraînement à la rétroaction électromyographique chez des anxieux chroniques. *Union Médicale du Canada*, **106**, 1530–1533.

Lavallée, Y. J., Lamontagne, Y., Annable, L., and Fontaine, F. (1980) *Characteristics of chronic anxious patients responding to EMG feedback training* (submitted for publication).

Marcus, N., and Levin, G. (1977) Clinical applications of biofeedback: implications for psychiatry. *Hospital and Community Psychiatry*, **28**, 21–25.

Nigl, A. J., and Jackson, B. (1979) Electromyograph biofeedback as an adjunct to standard psychiatric treatment. *Journal of Clinical Psychiatry*, **40**, 433–436.

Raskin, M., Johnson, G., and Rondestvedt, J. W. (1973) Chronic anxiety treated by feedback induced muscle relaxation. *Archives of General Psychiatry*, **28**, 263–267.

Raskin, M., Bali, L. R., and Peeke, H. V. (1980) Muscle biofeedback and transcendental meditation. *Archives of General Psychiatry*, **37**, 93–97.

Schultz, J. H. (1960) *Le training autogène*. Presses Universitaires de France, Paris.

Steffen, J. J. (1975) Electromyographically induced relaxation in the treatment of chronic alcohol abuse. *Journal of Consulting and Clinical Psychology*, **43**, 275.

Stoyva, J. (1975) La réponse de combat ou de fuite peut-elle être modifiée? in Trudel, G., and Lamontagne, Y. (eds.), *Modification du comportement en milieu clinique et en éducation*. Association des spécialistes en modification du comportement, Montréal, pp. 19–26.

AUTHOR INDEX

251

SUBJECT INDEX

259